inside bodybuilding

jim murray

 Contemporary Books, Inc.
Chicago

Library of Congress Cataloging in Publication Data

Murray, Jim.
    Inside bodybuilding.

    Includes index.
    1. Weight lifting.   I. Title.
GV546.M84   1978   796.4'1   77-91166
ISBN 0-8092-7725-5
ISBN 0-8092-7724-7 pbk.

Published by Contemporary Books, Inc.
180 North Michigan Avenue, Chicago, Illinois 60601
Manufactured in the United States of America
Library of Congress Catalog Card Number: 77-91166
International Standard Book Number: 0-8092-7725-5 (cloth)
                                    0-8092-7724-7 (paper)

Published simultaneously in Canada by
Beaverbooks
953 Dillingham Road
Pickering, Ontario L1W 1Z7
Canada

contents

acknowledgments

A number of people have been most cooperative and helpful in providing material for this book. John Grimek, Bill Pearl, and Boyer Coe were kind enough to allow me to use posed individual photographs, and John also provided photos previously published in *Strength & Health* magazine. Joe and Ben Weider provided the photos credited to the I. F. B. B., which previously were published in *Muscle Builder/Power* magazine. Don Prowant, of Levittown, Pennsylvania, took most of the exercise photos of Bob Cappiello, and T. J. Klein photographed Bob using the leg and lat machines. Bob Cappiello proved to be a true friend with endurance to match his muscles as he posed for all the pictures by Don in one sweat-soaked session. Al Raws took the picture of Nancy Borden and Bob Smith. The cover picture of Boyer Coe instructing Dave Galliano was taken by Theron Larroquette, and the exercise photos of Boyer were taken by Leonard Sirmopoulos, Convention Photography Studio. And my wife, Jane, was her usual cheerful, reliable self despite my cantankerous nit-picking over her typing of the manuscript.

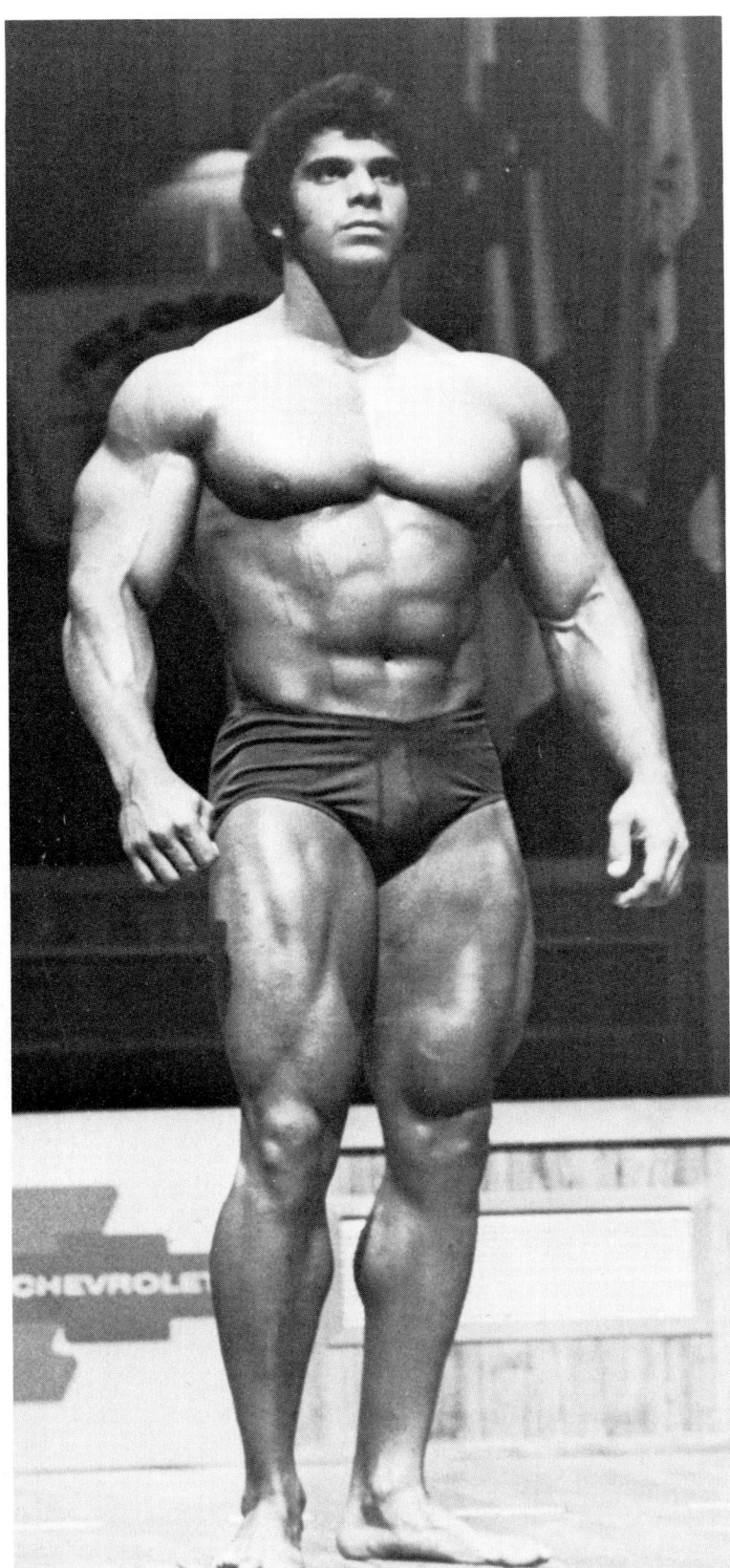

LOU FERRIGNO demonstrated that bodybuilders have muscles but are not "muscle-bound" with his versatile performance in the all-around athletic tests that comprise the televised "Superstars" competition. The 6′ 5″ Ferrigno, weighing more than 250 pounds, was especially outstanding at rowing, bicycling, weight lifting, and baseball hitting. (Photo courtesy IFBB)

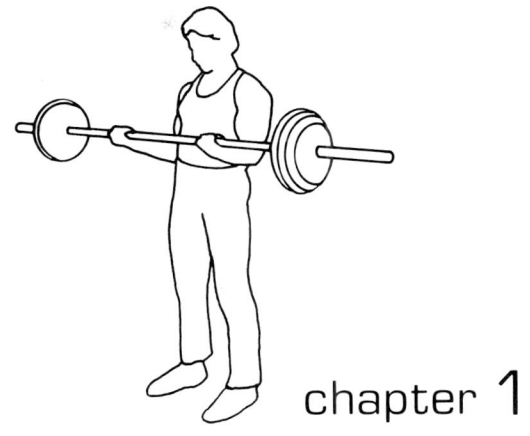

chapter 1

BODYBUILDING FACTS AND FICTION

Bodybuilding can be either a minor hobby, taking up about three hours a week of your time, or a highly competitive sport that calls for two to four hours of daily preparation and constant dietary discipline. It can produce a pleasant sensation of well-exercised muscles that feel taut and fit, or it can result in the agonized exhaustion of pumping to the absolute limit of strength and endurance.

Either way, there are attendant benefits to health and improved physical appearance. Anyone who thinks the end result of bodybuilding isn't improved appearance must believe that bodies like those of Laurel and Hardy look better than the bodies portrayed in classical sculpture.

You should realize at the outset that bodybuilding is highly individualized. What you get out of it depends upon two things: your natural endowments and how hard you are willing to work. This is true for both men and women since both sexes can use similar bodybuilding exercises to shape up and trim down.

Bodybuilding exercises tone all the muscles of the body. For both men and women this results in improved body shape, reduction of flabbiness, and a trimmer midsection. For men, because of hormonal differences, bodybuilding also results in larger muscles. How large a man's muscles get depends on his physical type and how hard he is willing to exercise.

PHYSICAL TYPES

Physical types are divided into three major categories, denoting leanness and fragility (ectomorphy), prominent muscles and bones (mesomorphy), and softness and fatness (endomorphy). No one is a 100 percent ectomorph, mesomorph, or endomorph, but the more mesomorphy present in a person's genetic makeup, the more muscle that person can develop by bodybuilding. The three physical types are rated on a scale of one to seven in each component, and it is most unlikely that anyone rating less than five in mesomorphy could ever become a champion bodybuilder in major contests. It also would be very difficult to overcome large ectomorphic or endomorphic components to become a champion bodybuilder, but a person rating six or seven in mesomorphy might do so if the ectomorphic or endomorphic component were no higher than three or four. A person who rated six or seven in mesomorphy would have a particular advantage in bodybuilding if he were a one in endomorphy and a two or three in ectomorphy because he easily could build muscle and yet remain lean with little tendency to take on fat.

Most people are intermediate physical types, and those who tend to be somewhat mesomorphic almost invariably are attracted to physical exercise. Mesomorphs like to feel their muscles working against a challenge. Those who are quick and aggressive gravitate to rough contact sports, while those who are competitive but not as aggressive tend to wind up in strenuous non-contact sports. Bodybuilding is one of these sports. Often, bodybuilding is combined successfully with a rough contact sport, especially football or one of the martial arts.

WHAT CAN BODYBUILDING DO FOR YOU?

Many people are active in bodybuilding simply for the reason that they want to look better. This is certainly a worthwhile goal. Not only does it denote a healthy self-esteem but it also improves the at-

tractiveness of the environment for the rest of us! Often, this self-improvement means only some trimming of the midsection for men and women and some building up of the shoulders and arms for men. Others are more ambitious, however. Some women seek to mold their bodies into shapely curves, and some men seek complete development of every muscle. When a man is sufficiently dedicated to undergo the self-discipline of regular exercise and constant attention to diet and also has the right combination of mesomorphic dominance over endomorphy and ectomorphy, he has the potential to become a bodybuilding champion. This may mean winning a "Mr. Hometown" contest, a state title, one of the major awards, such as Mr. America, Mr. U. S. A., Mr. Universe, or Mr. Olympia.

Some Myths Exploded

I often am amused by men who express concern that their muscles will get "too big" if they try a little bodybuilding exercise. They have nothing to fear! Practicing a few bodybuilding exercises does not set in motion a runaway process that inevitably produces a Mr. America body. If only it did! Hundreds of thousands of underweight or flabby young men would be delighted! In fact, some trimming of the midsection and increased muscle around the upper torso should be noticeable in a month to six weeks, but it takes at least a year to approach the kind of development required to win a contest, even for a natural mesomorph.

Another fear expressed by the would-be bodybuilder is that the activity will make him "muscle-bound." This will not happen. Bodybuilding will make the muscles larger and stronger, but as long as all the muscles are exercised—both extensors and flexors, for example, as opposed to only flexors—there will be no restriction of movement. If a person wants to acquire skill in a certain sport, however, he shouldn't expect bodybuilding to provide it. Bodybuilding exercises will help with general conditioning, but if you want to be a skilled tennis player, you have to play tennis.

Alex Aronis

There are many examples available to show that bodybuilding exercises do not handicap athletic performance. One individual who impressed me almost 30 years ago was a young man named Alex Aronis, who was featured in bodybuilding magazines for having developed an 18-inch arm at the age of 18. It happened that Aronis also was very bright and a good football player. He matriculated at the Naval Academy and, though not large at approximately 5'8" and 185 pounds, he was a star guard on the Navy "football team called desire." That team went on after a successful regular season (they were ranked fifth by UPI) against top-flight opposition to defeat a fine Mississippi team 21-0 in the Sugar Bowl on New Year's Day, 1956.

Lou Ferrigno

A more recent example was provided by Lou Ferrigno, winner of Mr. America and Mr. Universe titles and certainly representative of advanced bodybuilding training. If anyone was destined to be "muscle-bound," Lou should have been. Due to a hearing impairment, he had been prevented from taking part in the variety of sports for which his 6'5" frame and mesomorphic body structure otherwise would have qualified him. Instead, Ferrigno specialized in bodybuilding, with spectacular results, building up to well over 250 pounds of massive muscles.

When Lou Ferrigno was invited to appear in the nationally televised "Super-stars" competition against leading athletes from all major sports, he acquitted himself so well that he must have quieted for all time the myth that a bodybuilding specialist can't do anything but display his muscles. No one was greatly surprised when the powerful-appearing young man lifted a 300-pound barbell overhead or even when he proved outstanding at rowing. His broad back and muscular arms looked well-prepared for rowing and lifting. But when Lou also proved to be one of the best at bicycle racing—calling for speed and stamina—and also was outstanding in baseball hitting—attesting to his coordination and quick reflexes—television viewers must have had second thoughts about the supposed clumsiness and slowness of bodybuilders.

Bodybuilding in Athletic Training Programs

Aside from examples of advanced bodybuilders who exhibit a variety of athletic skills, it is noteworthy that the two key bodybuilding exercises—the bench press and the squat—are used almost universally in athletic training programs. There are few indeed in professional football who have not done bench presses with 200 to 300 pounds or more and who have not done squats with even heavier weights. Bill Toomey, former decathlon world-record holder and Olympic champion, could bench press more than 300 pounds while weighing only 190. Decathlon champions such as Toomey and Bruce Jenner developed fine physiques by training with weights but did not become as massively muscled as bodybuilders because they also spent many training hours running and practicing the demanding skills of the ten events in their specialty.

A man who wanted to emulate the physique of a decathlon athlete could do so—assuming a similar body type—by practicing bodybuilding exercises three days a week and jogging or running on three alternate days. These activities will produce similar physique results without requiring the exerciser to learn the decathlon skills.

CAN MUSCLE TURN TO FAT?

Another old wives' tale often heard about bodybuilding is that muscles developed to great size by exercise promptly turn into blobs of fat when the bodybuilder ceases training. This is no more true than the generalization that all athletes get fat when they stop participating in sports. First of all, muscle tissue is distinctly different from fat. One does not "turn into" the other. If a person has good muscle development due to exercise, he will lose some of it if he stops working out. The process can be seen in an arm or a leg that is placed in a cast as a result of injury. The confined muscles do not turn into fat; they atrophy (shrink).

If a bodybuilder stops exercising, he will begin to lose muscle size and strength, just as a runner will lose muscle size and strength in his legs if he stops running. Whether or not he replaces the muscle with fat depends upon his body type (somatotype) and his diet. A person who consumes no more food than his body needs for day-to-day activities (roughly 15 calories per pound of body weight, with individual variations) will not add fat. In fact, he is likely to lose weight as long as his intake does not exceed his needs because he will lose some solid muscle mass as a result of inactivity.

What happens to the non-training bodybuilder also depends on his somatotype; he will tend to revert to the physical type he would have been if he had not exercised. An inactive mesomorph with a large endomorphic component will put on fat unless he watches his diet carefully.

On the other hand, an inactive mesomorph with a large ectomorphic component will tend to lose weight and size.

The main point is this: people do not get fat because they formerly engaged in bodybuilding. They get fat because they are taking in more calories in food than they are expending in activity. The best evidence of this can be seen in the great number of obese people who have never done any bodybuilding. It is doubly unfortunate that these fat people have not done bodybuilding, incidentally, because if they had, chances are that their overweight bodies would at least have better proportions.

It is difficult to find an advanced bodybuilder who later has become truly obese. When these men give up or moderate their training (few ever give it up entirely), they may look a bit smoother and put on a few pounds, but by ordinary standards their proportions are still far superior to those of non-exercisers.

BODYBUILDING HAS NO AGE LIMITS

One of the great merits of bodybuilding is that it does not have to be discontinued as do so many competitive sports. Even if a former competitive bodybuilder loses interest in the long, intensive gym workouts and the rigid dietary discipline, he can stay in good shape by doing a few key exercises at home with an investment of no more than $100 to $200 in equipment. Unlike a pair of $25 jogging shoes, bodybuilding equipment—a barbell, pair of dumbbells, squat stands, and a bench—will never wear out. The initial investment will last a lifetime. I often am amused by claims that jogging is inexpensive as I see more serious joggers wearing out $50 to $100 worth of shoes a year while I continue to exercise with the old set of weights my parents gave me as a gift on my fourteenth birthday in 1940.

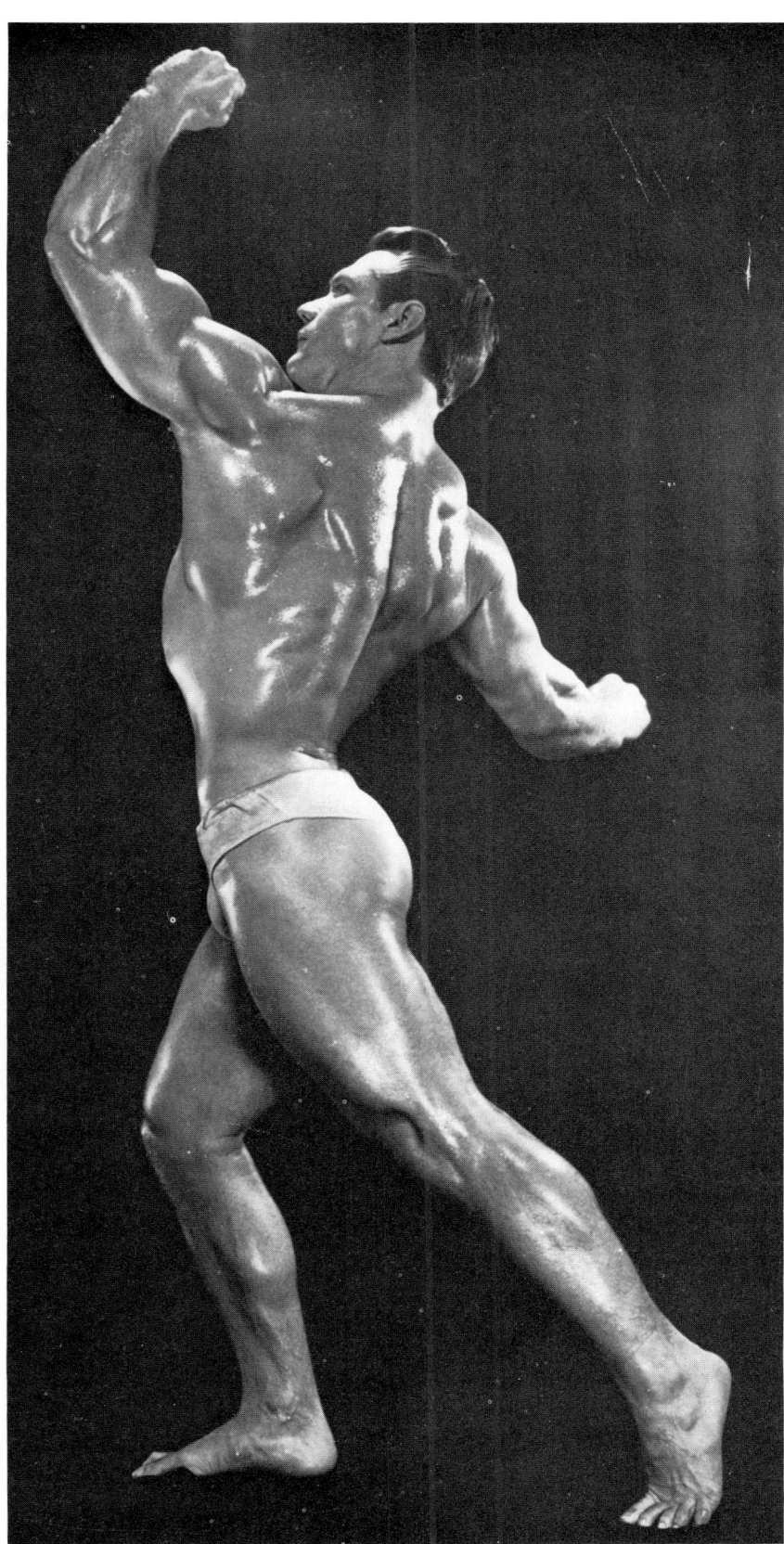

MASSIVELY MUSCLED JOHN GRIMEK dominated bodybuilding competition during the 1940–1950 decade. Although he retired from competition at age 40, Grimek continued to exercise to keep in shape. The photo on page 6 shows him at 58. (Photos provided by John C. Grimek)

Sig Klein

A number of "old-timers" in bodybuilding still keep in fine shape, showing that minimal physical deterioration occurs if a person continues to exercise. An outstanding example is Siegmund Klein, who was noted for his physique and strength shortly after World War I and who continued to operate a fine gymnasium in New York City until well past ordinary retirement age. When Sig finally disposed of the studio on Seventh Avenue where he had taught exercise to many stars of stage and screen, he didn't really retire. Instead, he continued to instruct part time at another health club when well into his seventies. Arnold Schwarzenegger, in his late twenties and at his physical prime, shortly after winning Mr. Universe and Mr. Olympia titles and starring in the movie "Pumping Iron," was impressed by the fact that Sig had been able to go through an entire workout with him. Sig used lighter weights, of course; aside from being more than 40 years older than Arnold, he was some 60 or 70 pounds lighter. Sig's weight never varied much from the 150 pounds he weighed in his heyday as a competing strongman.

John Grimek

Another remarkable example of an "old-timer" who never seemed to age was John Grimek. John was a versatile strongman-athlete, having won national weight lifting titles and representing the United States on the 1936 Olympic team before winning Mr. America titles in 1940 and 1941. John was already 31 when he won his second Mr. America title (at which time a rule was passed that a winner could no longer succeed himself because it appeared that he might come back and collect a trophy every year), an age when many men consider themselves too old to do anything strenuous. It was only a beginning for Grimek, however, who went on to defeat such notable (and younger) Mr. America winners as Clarence Ross and Steve Reeves (of movie Hercules fame) in Mr. U. S. A. and Mr. Universe competition.

Grimek finally gave up active competition in 1949, but he never stopped exer-

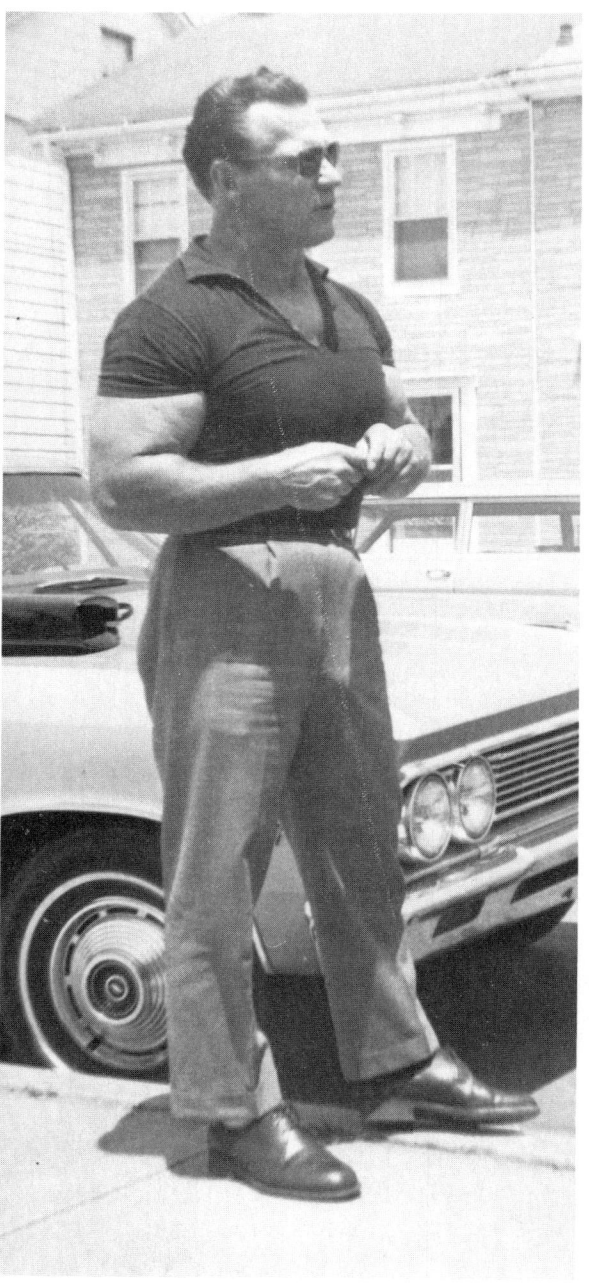

cising. I often had the pleasure of working out with John when we were co-editors of *Strength & Health* magazine in the early 1950s. I often was astounded to see this man, in his forties, easily perform high-repetition dumbbell presses with 100 pounds in each hand and up to 20 consecutive squats with about 300 pounds on legs that seemed to belong to a man half his age. Then a number of years passed during which I didn't see John. One day, a business trip took me through his home town of York, PA, and I dropped in for a visit. It was as though I had passed through a time warp. There was John, still editing the magazine—and still packing a pair of massively muscled arms, powerful shoulders, deep chest, and amazingly small waist. He still looked only fortyish and had the body of a well-trained athlete of 30. I could have walked out the door one day and returned the next, but in the meantime, John had become chronologically old enough to collect Social Security! Unbelievably, this vigorous, enthusiastic, ageless superman had turned 65!

Fountain of Youth?

The youth-preserving effect of bodybuilding may not work for everyone as it did for Klein and Grimek, but they are not the only examples of this effect. Roy Hilligenn, who was the 1951 Mr. America, competed impressively in the 1976 Mr. Universe contest at 54. Pictures taken of him in 1951 and 1976 could have been snapped on the same day.

Several well-known gym operators have maintained superb, ageless physiques into their forties. Bill Pearl won his final Mr. Universe contest at 41 before retiring from active competition to devote full time to his Physical Fitness Architects and Pasadena (California) Health Club businesses. Ed Corney, who is pictured on the cover of Charles Gaines's and George Butler's best seller, *Pumping Iron*, continued to compete successfully in major international physique contests in his mid-forties.

Other gym operators who have made good use of their own facilities to hold time at bay are Vince Gironda and Joe Nista. Fifty is just another year to men such as these.

PHYSIOLOGICAL EFFECTS

What is it about this form of exercise that allows aging men to retain bodies that look more youthful than the bodies of average men 20 years younger? No one knows at the present time, and it may be just that these natural mesomorphs have found the activity formula that works best for their body types.

On the other hand, there may be some special physiological effect of bodybuilding that hasn't yet been identified. The slender, wiry types that predominate in physiology labs tend to dismiss bodybuilding as an activity that merely builds muscle but does nothing for health. It does do more than build muscle, however, as Dr. Fred Abbo found out. Dr. Abbo conducted a study of the effects of various kinds of exercise on the body's natural production of steroids. Dr. Abbo's results, presented at a Midwest regional meeting of the American College of Sports Medicine, were reported in *Medical Tribune* on May 4, 1966, page 29.

It previously had been determined that the average ratio of 17-ketosteroids (17-KS) to 17-hydroxycorticosteroids (17-OHCS) in normally healthy 20-year-old men was 2.0. With aging, over a period from 20 to 80 years, the ratio progressively declines. With a baseline established, Dr. Abbo studied 49 non-obese men aged 37 to 54 whose primary exercise consisted of handball, calisthenics, running, and swimming and compared the results with those obtained on 26 men in the same age range whose primary exercise was weight training. Aside from their hobby exercises, the men in both groups led sedentary lives. Dr. Abbo found that 14 percent of the men who trained on endurance exercises had 17-KS/17-OHCS ratios greater than 2.0 (the "youthful" level). By contrast, a full 42 percent of the weight-trained men had ratios greater than the 2.0 found normal in healthy 20-year-olds.

Investigating further, Dr. Abbo studied a 40-year-old man over a period of 16 months. At first, the man exercised intermittently, but then he stepped up to intensive and regular running of one or two miles from three to five times a week. He also did calisthenics. Finally, the man added weight training to his program for the last four months. The subject's 17-KS/17-OHCS ratio was essentially unchanged during the 12 months of running and calisthenics, but when he added exercise with weights, the "youthful" 2.0 ratio was achieved. Dr. Abbo was not prepared to claim these results definitely established a special value for weight training, but he did conclude that they provide support for the usefulness of this type of exercise.

Incidentally, the role of bodybuilding in making people look more youthful is not confined to men. Doris Barrilleaux of Florida regularly practices bodybuilding exercises at 46 and has a better figure than most women 20 years younger.

BODYBUILDING AND YOUR HEART

The negative attitude of many physiologists toward bodybuilding appears to be based on the belief that it does not benefit the cardiovascular system. This belief is questionable. There is no doubt that such exercises as jogging and cycling do have positive effects on the cardiovascular system, as judged by the tests used by physiologists, so anyone seeking only cardiovascular fitness can be advised to jog or ride a bicycle. Jogging and cycling definitely do not do as much to develop all the muscles of the body as bodybuilding does, however. So if there are more general benefits from bodybuilding, it does not seem fair to dismiss it as "merely" a muscle-builder.

Cardiovascular Training

There is evidence, too, that bodybuilding does have—or can be practiced to have—a cardiovascular training effect. To produce a training effect on the cardiovascular system, physiologists believe, it is necessary to exercise at an intensity that raises the pulse rate to approximately 70 percent of its maximum, a rate that decreases with age. Seventy percent for people in normal health would be 140 beats per minute at age 20–25, 136 at 30, 128 at 40, 124 at 45, 119 at 50, 115 at 55, 111 at 60, and 107 at 65. You can calculate your "normal maximum" by subtracting your age from 220. If you have any doubt about your fitness to exercise at an increased heart rate, you should have a medical examination first.

In bodybuilding, if you perform a set of ten repetitions of an exercise such as the squat, your pulse rate is most likely to increase to the 70 percent-of-maximum level or more. To maintain this elevated pulse rate, you must minimize the rest periods between sets. Because the work done in a bodybuilding exercise is intense, the natural tendency is to rest until you feel comfortably ready to resume. But if you seek a conditioning effect as well as increased muscle size and strength, you should limit the rest period between sets.

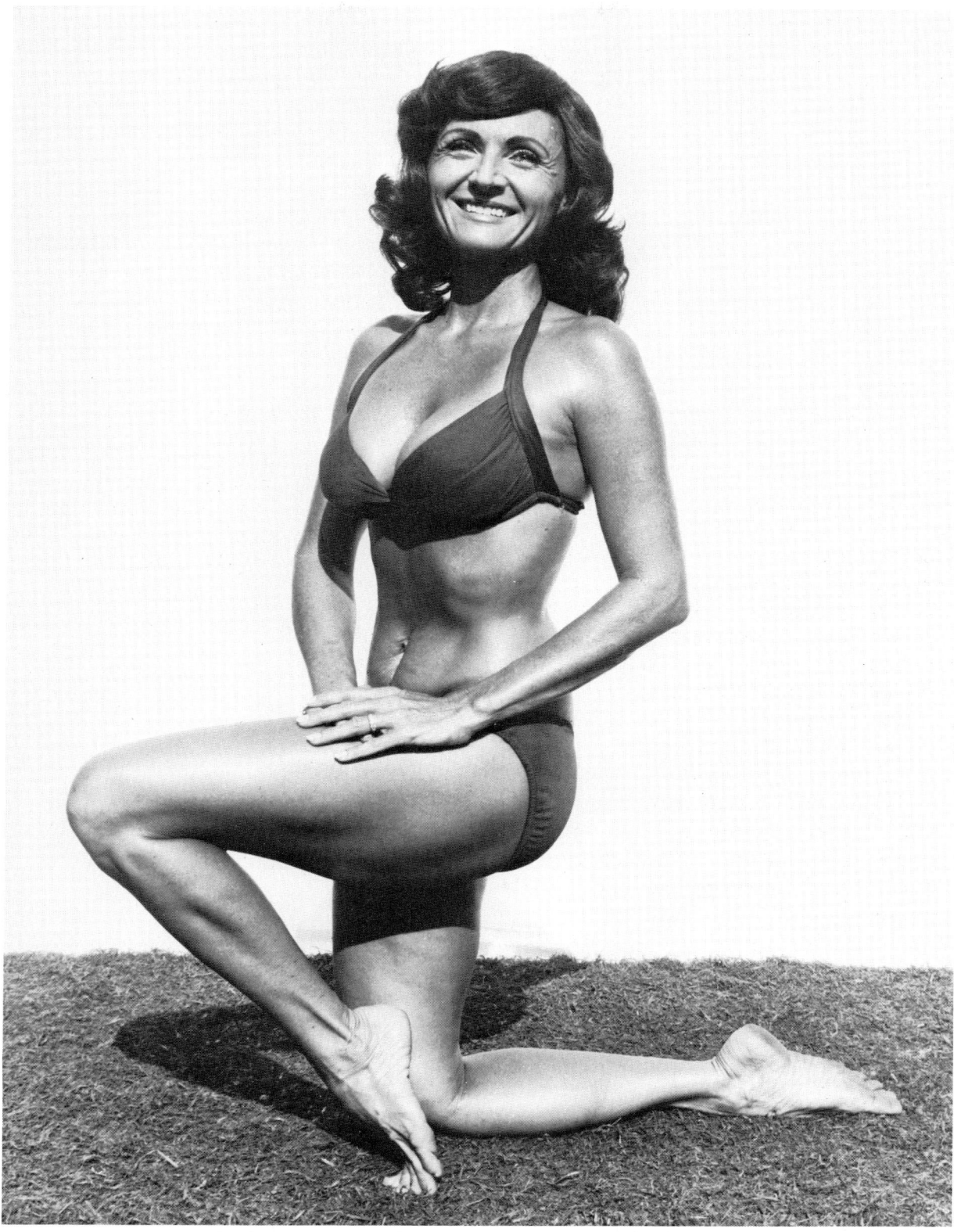

DORIS BARRILLEAUX is living proof that bodybuilding does not develop lumpy muscles on normal women. She also is good evidence that long-term practice of bodybuilding maintains vitality and shapeliness for women past 40. Doris, 46, has been bodybuilding for 30 years with obviously beneficial effects. (Photo by Dick Falcon)

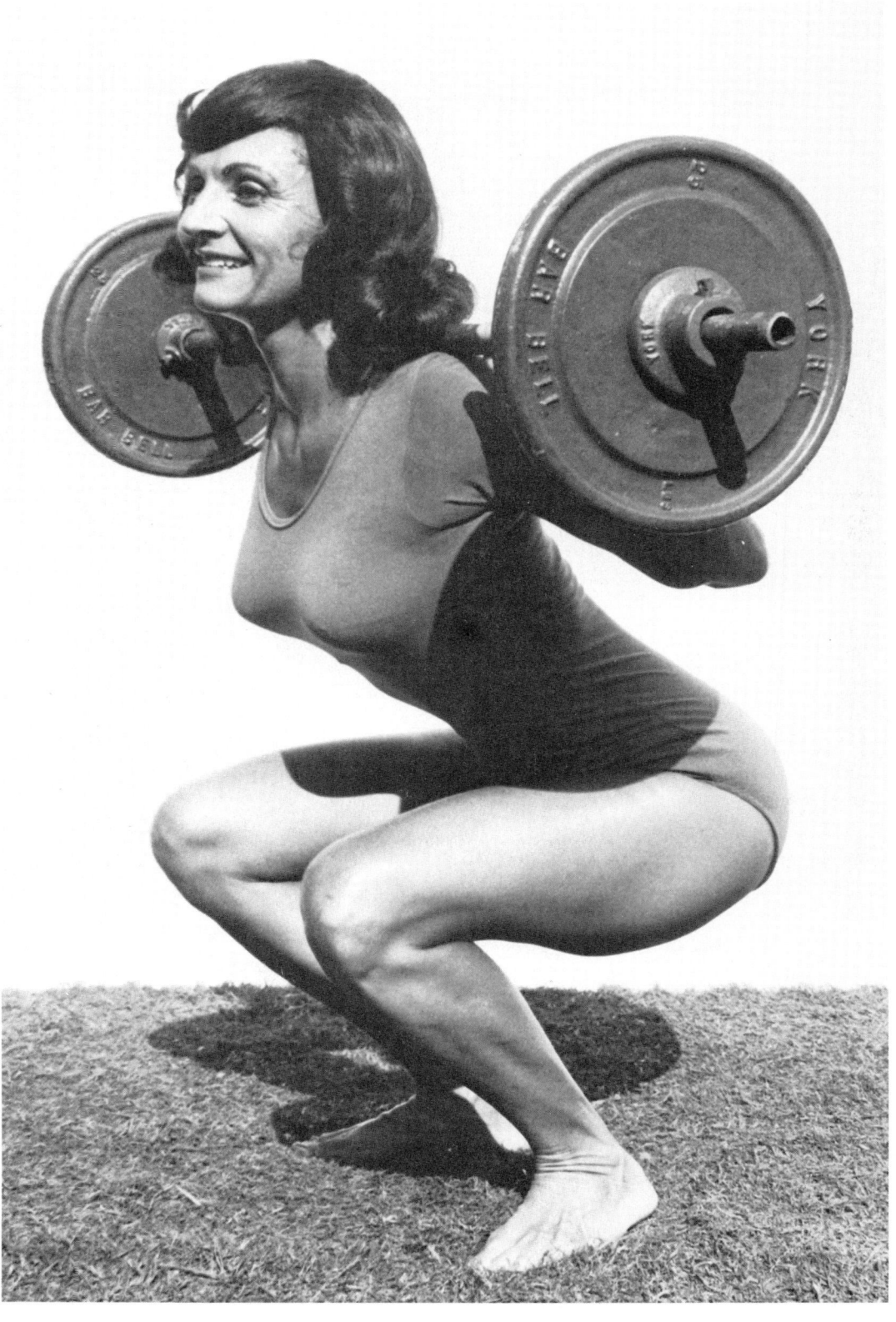

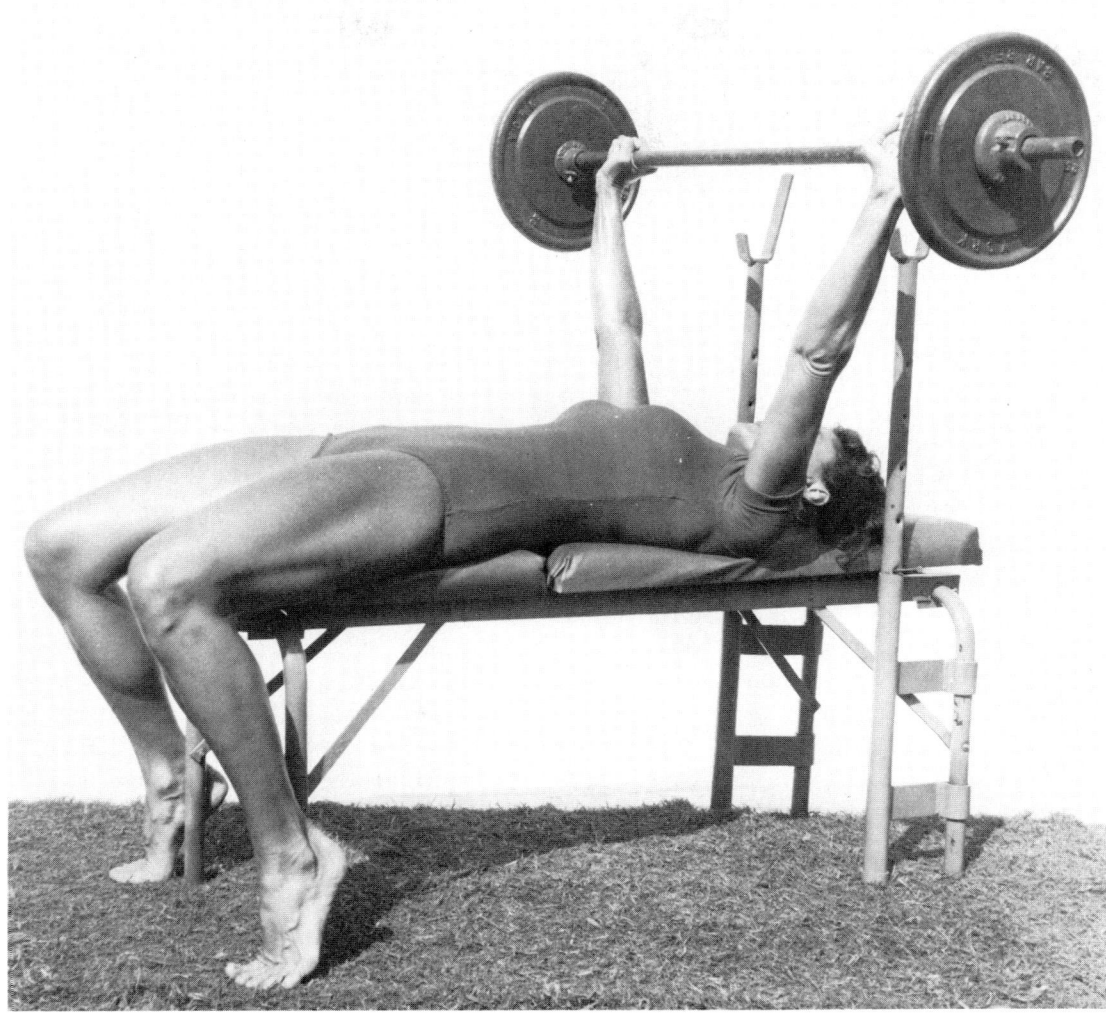

An Exercising Routine

For example, you might do three sets of squats, each set followed by a set of pullovers. For one week, you might allow yourself 1½ minutes for rest between sets. The second week you would reduce the rest between sets to 1¼ minutes. The third week you would reduce the rest to 1 minute, the fourth week, to 45 seconds, and the fifth week, to 30 seconds. Such an approach calls for gradual reduction of rest breaks, with monitoring of your pulse between exercises. If you find that your pulse is elevated above 70 percent of maximum and that it does not slow to 70 percent of maximum in the allotted time, you can extend the rest break to the time it does take for your pulse to return to the target rate. The idea is to take just enough rest so that your pulse rate slows down to near the 70 percent-of-maximum level, and then do another set of the exercise or begin the next exercise in your routine.

This approach has been used in weight

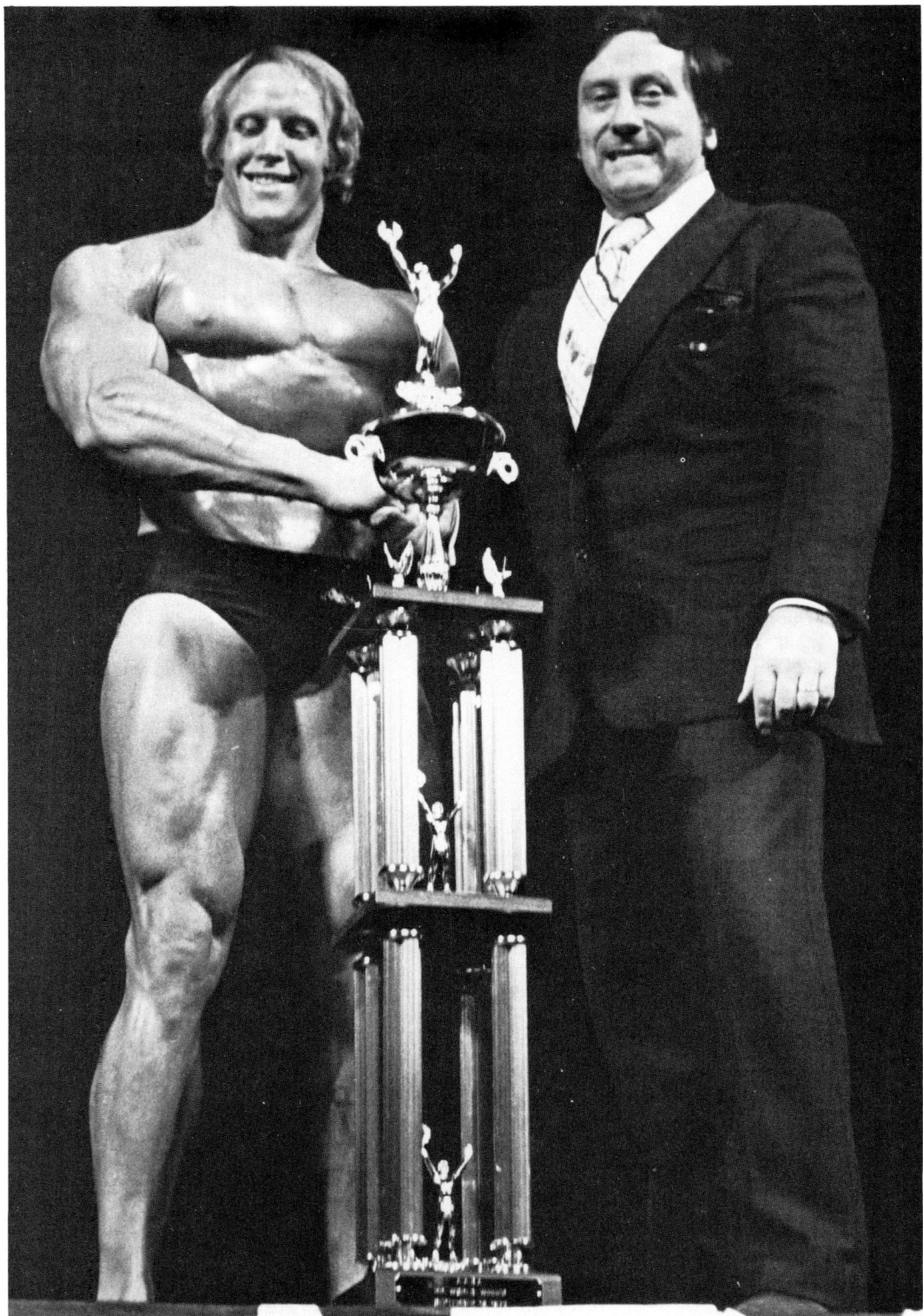

FORMERLY A PROFESSIONAL football player with the New York Jets, Mike Katz showed "high-good" to "superior" fitness on a standard battery of physical fitness tests conducted at a university physiology laboratory. Katz, shown receiving a major award from bodybuilding patron Joe Weider, was tested after he had undergone intensive training for the Mr. Universe contest. (Photo courtesy IFBB)

training for athletic conditioning—bursts of exercise with minimal rest breaks, going from one exercise to the next—and its application is called "circuit training." It is used by many champion bodybuilders for another reason as well: when the muscles are repeatedly taxed by difficult exercise, they are pumped with oxygenated blood and growth is stimulated. Regardless of the motive, the physiological effect has to be the same.

Mike Katz

Charles Gaines and George Butler reported in their book, *Pumping Iron*, that tests for cardiovascular fitness on Mike Katz, a 6'1", 240-pound Mr. America and Mr. World titlist, produced "spectacular" results. The tests, done by Dr. Larry Golding of Kent State University, measured Mike's physical work capacity on a stationary bicycle of the type used in physiology laboratories. The big bodybuilder, a man with a 52" chest, 20" arms, and 26" thighs, tested to a maximum work load of 2,400 KPM, a rating that was clear off the scale used to measure physical work capacity.

Mike Katz had been an outstanding football player as well as a bodybuilder, good enough to play as a professional for the New York Jets. But it was bodybuilding, not football, that was responsible for his "high-good" on one test (heart rate, sitting) to "superior" on the rest of the battery of aerobic tests for cardiovascular fitness, for he had just completed weeks of concentrated bodybuilding workouts to prepare for a Mr. Universe contest. In view of this, how can anyone seriously criticize bodybuilding for not contributing to cardiovascular conditioning?

Jim Lorimer, an attorney who practices bodybuilding as a hobby and who co-promoted Mr. Olympia contests with six-time titlist Arnold Schwarzenegger, likens the proper approach in bodybuilding to a three-legged stool, which will tip over if any of its three legs is not balanced with the other two. The three legs are 1) increasing resistance in the exercises to build strength and muscle; 2) repeated sets and a variety of exercises for shape and definition; and 3) limited rest pauses between sets and exercises for cardiovascular effect and general conditioning.

A number of bodybuilders, incidentally, do practice fast jogging or slow running, as much to burn off fat and increase muscularity as for health benefits. The main goal of the competitive bodybuilder is a muscular appearance; the fact that he also becomes fit is coincidental.

WHERE TO GO on a date? How about your local health club for a fitness-promoting bodybuilding workout. Nancy Borden, shown performing leg extensions, and Bob Smith, incline-pressing heavy dumbbells, are University of Delaware grads who often start a fun weekend with a workout. (Photo by Al Raws)

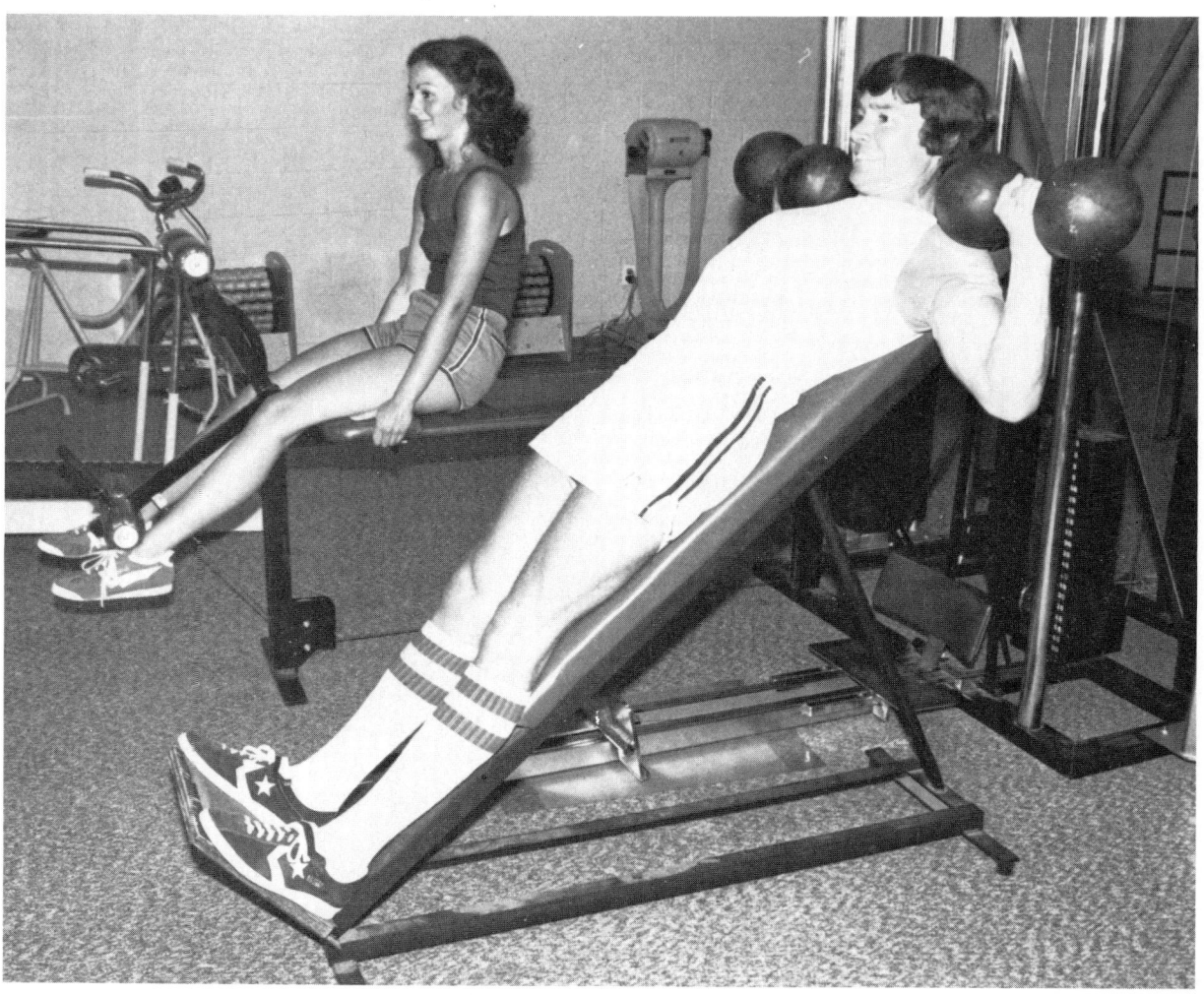

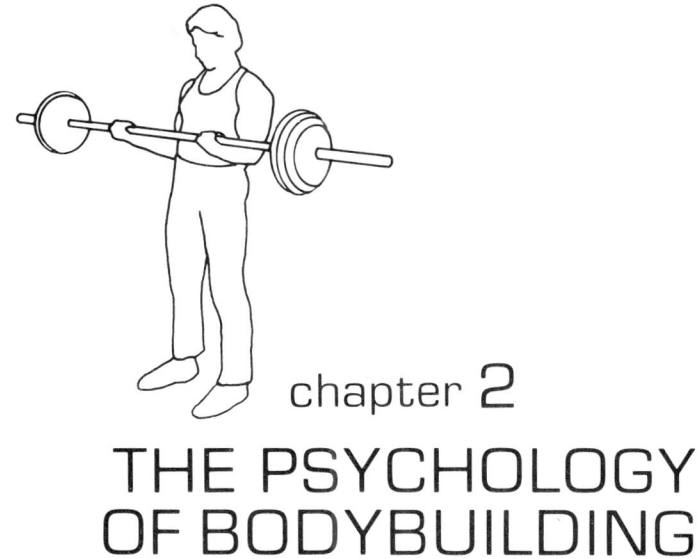

chapter 2

THE PSYCHOLOGY OF BODYBUILDING

People who comment on the psychology of bodybuilding tend to be non-bodybuilders, looking upon the successful bodybuilder as some sort of alien personality. The bodybuilder must be narcissistic, one might conclude; look at how concerned he is with his appearance. The bodybuilder must be insecure, another might surmise; note how concerned he is with developing large muscles. Actually, there are many kinds of narcissism. A lazier man than a bodybuilder might try to adorn his body with the latest fashions. This takes less effort than adding an inch to his biceps. Another insecure man might bolster his self-image by driving a sports car. In this way, the car can do the work, and he can be spared the time and effort needed for the sets of bench presses required to develop a big chest and broad shoulders.

But what of the non-bodybuilder's psyche? What is it about a well-muscled man that is so disturbing to some muscleless men and to those women who profess to be "turned off" by big muscles? Could it be that these people are intimidated—subtly frightened—by clearly visible evidence of superior physical development?

People who express admiration for classical sculpture, such as the Farnese Hercules, paradoxically recoil at the sight of a living man who is as well-muscled as the statue. Perhaps it is time for some mesomorphic psychologist to study the reasons why some people feel so threatened by a well-muscled man.

Suppose a young man does compensate

for feelings of inferiority by exercising to develop large muscles. Is this any more reprehensible than compensating by clawing his way to the top in business or developing a large bankroll?

THE BODYBUILDER'S PERSONALITY

Dr. Peter Karpovich, the famed research physiologist, commented in a book we co-authored many years ago: "Even if a young Hercules does proudly strut when he is in the field of vision of young damsels, or even of weak, flabby, obese, and otherwise discreditable samples of the male of our species, can you blame him very much?" In the book, *Weight Training in Athletics* (Prentice-Hall, 1956), Dr. Karpovich pointed out that acquired ugliness of the body often results from neglect by its owner. Such ugliness is unnecessary; it can be prevented or corrected by bodybuilding exercises.

There are those who seem to want to believe that bodybuilders lack a normal interest in the opposite sex. This belief is so ridiculous as to deserve little comment. It may be possible to find evidence of some isolated aberrant behavior, but it certainly isn't the rule. All one has to do to determine the heterosexuality of bodybuilders is to check on the champions in the sport who are married with families.

From first-hand observation of many outstanding bodybuilders as well as personal friendship with many who have won top national and international contests, I can testify that these men have personalities that are no "different" from other people who have compelling interests—from actors to professional athletes in various sports to skilled artisans to research scientists to successful businessmen. Every walk of life is represented by those who are quietly competent and unassuming as well as by those who are self-centered and arrogant.

Practicing bodybuilding exercises for hours is no more monotonous and self-centered than the gruelling training done by distance runners and swimmers, nor is it any more solitary and obsessive. The bodybuilder practices a greater variety of movements than does a distance runner or swimmer, and most relatively serious bodybuilders enjoy the camaraderie of workouts in a gym or health club with other people who have similar interests. Most of the people I've worked out with in weight training gyms have fun while they exercise, joking or conversing seriously with training partners and helping each other train. In fact, some of the more enlightened health clubs now encourage co-ed exercise facilities, adding to the socializing possibilities.

THE PRACTICE OF BODYBUILDING

The practice of bodybuilding is a seemingly simple but actually complex activity. Before you can attack its complexities, however, you must first understand the simple approach.

Bodybuilding is done by working muscles against resistance. In order to have a fully developed body, all the muscle groups must be worked. In order to have a well-proportioned body, the least developed and responsive muscles must be worked harder than those that grow easily. There are variations in individual response to exercise, but in general the best results are obtained by working against resistance (usually weight in the form of a barbell or dumbbell) that permits between 8 and 12 repetitions. If the weight is too heavy to permit 8 repetitions of an exercise without stopping to rest, it still will develop muscle size and shape and it will develop more sheer strength and power than exercising with less resistance, but it will not produce the full flush of blood to the working muscle that is referred to as "a good pump."

To get the good pump also requires concentration and, in some cases, a bit of technique. More about that later.

Exercising in "Sets"

In addition to working an individual muscle or related group of muscles between 8 and 12 repetitions, it is necessary to repeat the 8–12 repetitions several times (sets) with a brief rest after each set. The rest should be kept brief for two reasons: 1) the muscle-building pump effect is greater if it is not permitted to subside before additional work is done; 2) there is also a conditioning effect—a benefit to cardiovascular fitness—if the heart rate is not permitted to return to normal during a workout.

How many sets? That depends on how much work a given body part needs, how an individual responds to exercise, and how ambitious the exerciser is. Anyone can achieve improved contours, increased general fitness, and greater strength by doing three sets of eight to twelve repetitions of several key exercises.

For example, suppose you have no other equipment than a 100-pound barbell set. You can produce noticeable bodybuilding results by doing the following exercises. Curl the barbell from thighs to shoulders ten times with a weight that might permit one or two more repetitions than ten. Rest a minute and do ten (or nine or eight) more. Rest another minute and do at least eight more, trying for nine or ten. Then select a weight that you can not press overhead more than twelve times and do only ten presses. Rest a minute and do at least eight more. Take another rest and do another eight (or nine or ten if you can). You then will have done three sets of curls and three sets of presses. Just those two exercises, using enough weight to permit at least eight but

no more than twelve repetitions for three sets, are enough to improve greatly the strength and appearance of the arms and shoulders of a young man beyond the age of puberty.

How Many Sets Should You Do?

Many men who just want to keep in shape and build up their arms and shoulders a bit can do so with those two exercises plus twenty-five to fifty sit-ups and a mile of jogging three days a week— providing they have no unusual problems, such as excessive obesity.

The more ambitious bodybuilder will need a great deal more exercise than that, however. Even a naturally muscular (mesomorphic) person will need to perform resistance exercises for every part of the body in order to get superior results. And he will need to do more sets—five or six at least. The champion bodybuilders who compete in best-built-man contests think nothing of doing eight to ten sets of a single exercise for one body part during a workout.

Surprisingly, women can use a similar approach, doing the same basic exercises, though few women will be interested in doing more than three sets of an exercise unless they are training for power and muscular endurance to prepare for a competitive sport. Despite all the idealistic talk of equality, women will not be able to exercise with as much resistance as men. Some strong women may be able to match the strength of weak men, but they simply will not be able to keep up with strong men. The reason is that they lack male hormones. For the same reason, the same exercise that produces muscular bulges in men will produce only firm and attractive curves in women.

Equipment

The ideal way to practice bodybuilding is

to join a gymnasium or health club where a variety of equipment is available and where there are instructors or knowledgeable training partners to show you how or help motivate you. You can practice bodybuilding at home, however, with a minimal investment in equipment that will last a lifetime. The essential items include an adjustable barbell, a pair of adjustable dumbbells, squat racks, and a bench with uprights for supine pressing. Barbell/dumbbell combination sets cost from $40 to $60 and include weights for a 100-pound barbell plus a pair of 42½-pound dumbbells; $65 to $75 combination sets will enable you to load the barbell to 160 pounds. For $250 to $300 you can buy a 300-pound Olympic-type barbell and a pair of adjustable 42½-pound dumbbells. (The weighted discs or "plates" that adjust the poundage of an exercise set will not fit on an Olympic bar.) A pair of adjustable, shoulder-high squat stands costs about $40 to $60, and a bench with uprights costs between $35 and $50. These items are shown in the illustrations of exercises in this book. All-purpose exercise benches that will serve as squat stands, a flat-pressing bench, or an incline bench are available for about $100.

Many more exercises are possible with the specialized equipment available in gymnasiums (some of which is pictured throughout this book), but great physiques have been built with the four basic items described, and they certainly are adequate for the person who just wants to look and feel "a little better."

MUSCLE FOCUS

The next chapter will describe how to do exercises for every body part and how to arrange the exercises into effective bodybuilding routines.

But before getting into the individual exercises, it's worth pausing for a moment to consider a basic approach to all bodybuilding exercises. This book will describe how to perform the movements correctly, but you must learn for yourself how to *feel* the exercise working the muscles that you want to affect. For example, suppose you are doing the simple arm-flexing exercise called the curl that is used to develop the biceps muscles of the front of the upper arm. You simply can hold the weight at thigh level with arms straight and then bring the weight to your shoulder by bending your arms. That will have some bodybuilding effect, but it really isn't bodybuilding.

To get the full bodybuilding effect on the biceps, you must flex your arms deliberately, consciously contracting the biceps, and all the while *thinking* biceps. In a sense, you are contracting the biceps as you would if someone asked you to "show me your muscle." The weight goes along for the ride and provides the resistance needed to challenge the muscle fibers and make them grow.

Think about it. You move the weight, but that isn't what it's all about. What it's about is focusing on the muscle you want to develop, forcing it to respond, and molding it into the shape you want.

Champion bodybuilders seem to have two things going for them when they exercise. One is that their bodies have the right leverage and metabolism to build muscle, and the other is that they find the way to do the exercise that focuses the work on the muscle they want to build. Often, their natural structure combines with an instinctive feel for exercise so muscles grow no matter what the champions do. Many times, however, men who later develop prize-winning physiques have to experiment for months and years until they find the right combination of exercises, methods of performance, and special diets that take them to the top.

GETTING STARTED

This book can't begin to provide you with all the possible approaches, so it will concentrate on supplying enough basic information to get you started, along with details of how one bodybuilding champion prepares himself for top-level competition. If you become serious about bodybuilding competition, however, you will need to read the advice of many instructors as well as periodicals devoted to bodybuilding, exercise, and nutrition. Everything you read won't apply to you, so you'll have to study the subject intelligently, noting your individual responses and learning to make the best of them. You also will need to watch advanced bodybuilders in action to see how they perform the exercises.

As you read about and observe bodybuilders, you will come across some ideas that actually border on the bizarre. Some very strange training approaches have been advised because an individual with great potential is somewhat eccentric. This person succeeds in developing a lot of impressive-looking muscles despite ideas about training that might work for only a very few with comparable physical and psychological makeup. Often a champion succeeds as much in spite of what he does as because of it!

Gyms and Publications

Although several top bodybuilders have become outstanding instructors, many outstanding instructors have not had great personal success in competition. Some whose gyms you might want to visit or enroll in if you live nearby are Bill Pearl in Pasadena and Vince Gironda in North Hollywood, California, and Boyer Coe in Metairie, Louisiana. There are other gyms in metropolitan areas where outstanding bodybuilders congregate, such as Gold's in Santa Monica and the Mid-City gym in New York City. You can get an idea where other gyms are by reading articles about top physique men in magazines devoted to bodybuilding; the articles often mention various champions' favorite training haunts.

Among magazines that devote space to practical, applicable information on bodybuilding are:

Muscle Builder/Power
21100 Erwin Street
Woodland Hills, CA 91364

Muscular Development
P. O. Box 1707
York, PA 17405

Muscle Mag International
Unit One—270 Rutherford Road
Brampton, Ontario, Canada

Muscle Training Illustrated
1665 Utica Avenue
Brooklyn, NY 11234

Iron Man
512 Black Hills Avenue
Alliance, NE 69301

Strength & Health
P. O. Box 1707
York, PA 17405

LEG EXTENSIONS strengthen and define the thigh muscles. This exercise also can be done with weighted sandals but is more conveniently performed with special apparatus, as shown.

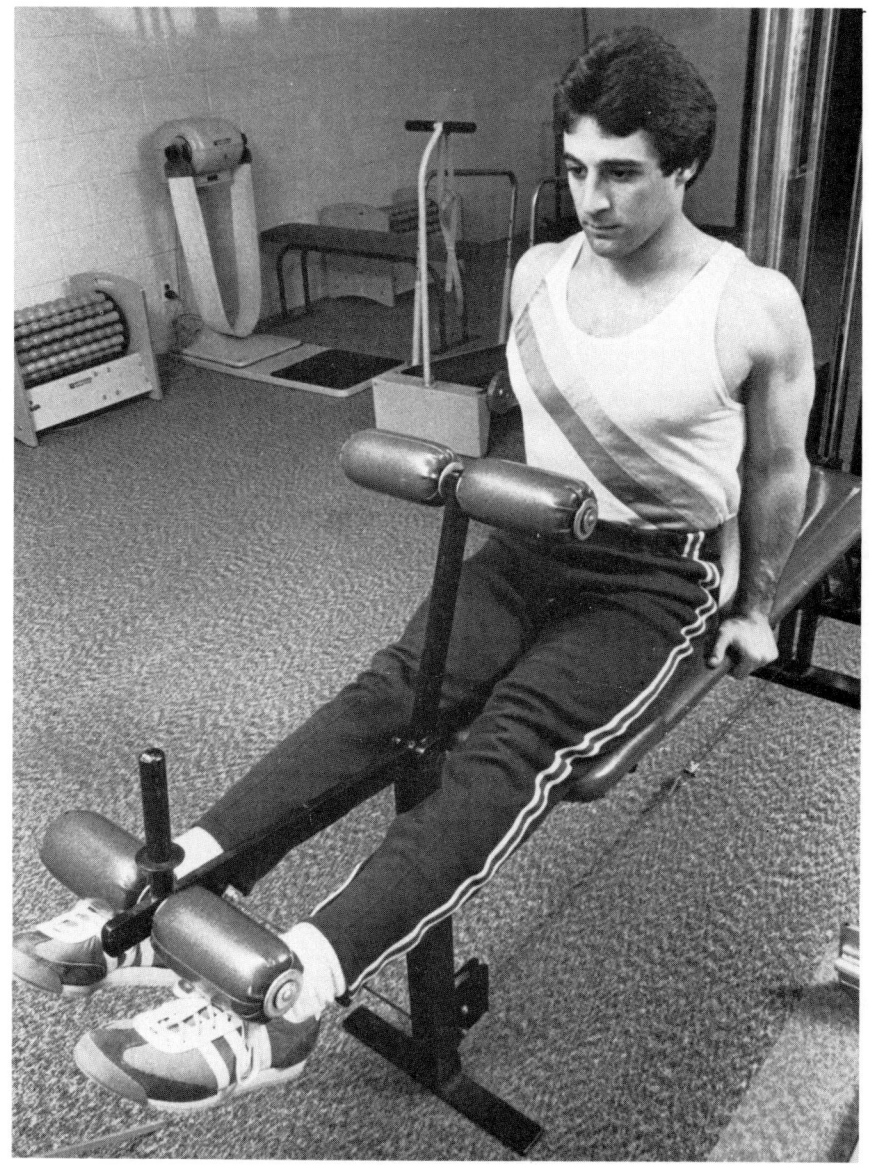

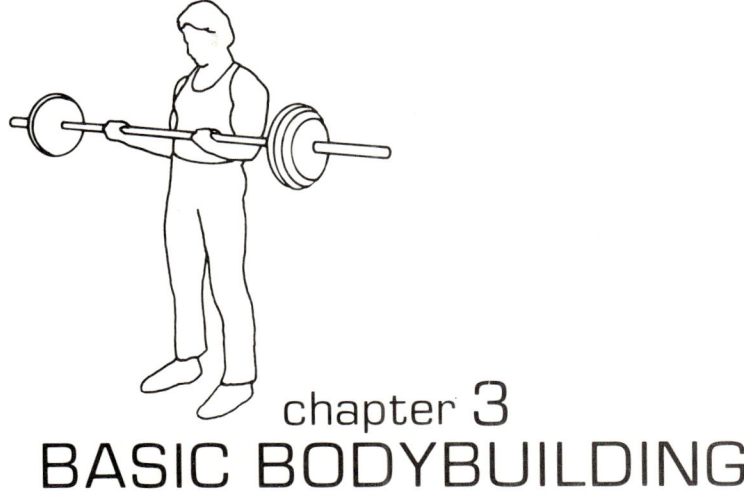

chapter 3
BASIC BODYBUILDING

Although it is possible for a young man to develop pleasing proportions by doing no more than barbell presses and curls, sit-ups, and some jogging, the proper way to approach bodybuilding is with an exercise routine that works all the muscles of the body. There is a tendency on the part of many beginners to concentrate on exercises for the body parts that they want most to develop—often the arms and shoulders—but, in fact, the arms and shoulders will respond better if the entire body is subjected to growth-building exercise.

The best approach to the sport for anyone but an advanced bodybuilder who is seriously preparing for a Mr. Best-Built-Man contest is to work out three times a week, on alternate days, with exercises for every part of the body in each of the three workouts. The following is a solid, basic routine for beginners:

1. Supine press on bench, 1 to 5 sets.

2. Squat, 1 to 5 sets.
3. Deep-breathing pullover, 1 to 5 sets.
4. Rowing exercise, 1 to 3 sets.
5. Curl, 1 to 3 sets.
6. Rise-on-toes, 1 to 3 sets.
7. Sit-up, 1 to 3 sets.
8. Press, 1 to 3 sets.

The supine press and squat are done first and second because they are key building exercises that permit use of heavy weights and jolt the body into muscular growth. They also take a lot of energy, so it's a good idea to do them while you're still fresh.

THE BENCH PRESS

First, the supine press on bench, better known as the "bench press." You will need a bench, with or without extended supports for the barbell. If you don't have a bench with supports, you will need a training partner to hand you the weight.

Begin the exercise by lying on the bench, feet on the floor, as in the illustrations, with the barbell at straight arms' length over your chest. Your hands should be spaced wider than your shoulders, about 20 to 30 inches apart, with an overhand grip. Take a deep breath and lower the weight smoothly, under control, to touch make you work, but not so hard that you couldn't do one or two more if you had to. Start your experimenting with weights that are obviously light and easy to handle. For women and young boys, this may be a total of 20 pounds, a 5-foot barbell handle and collars. For young men of average size, 40 pounds is a good weight

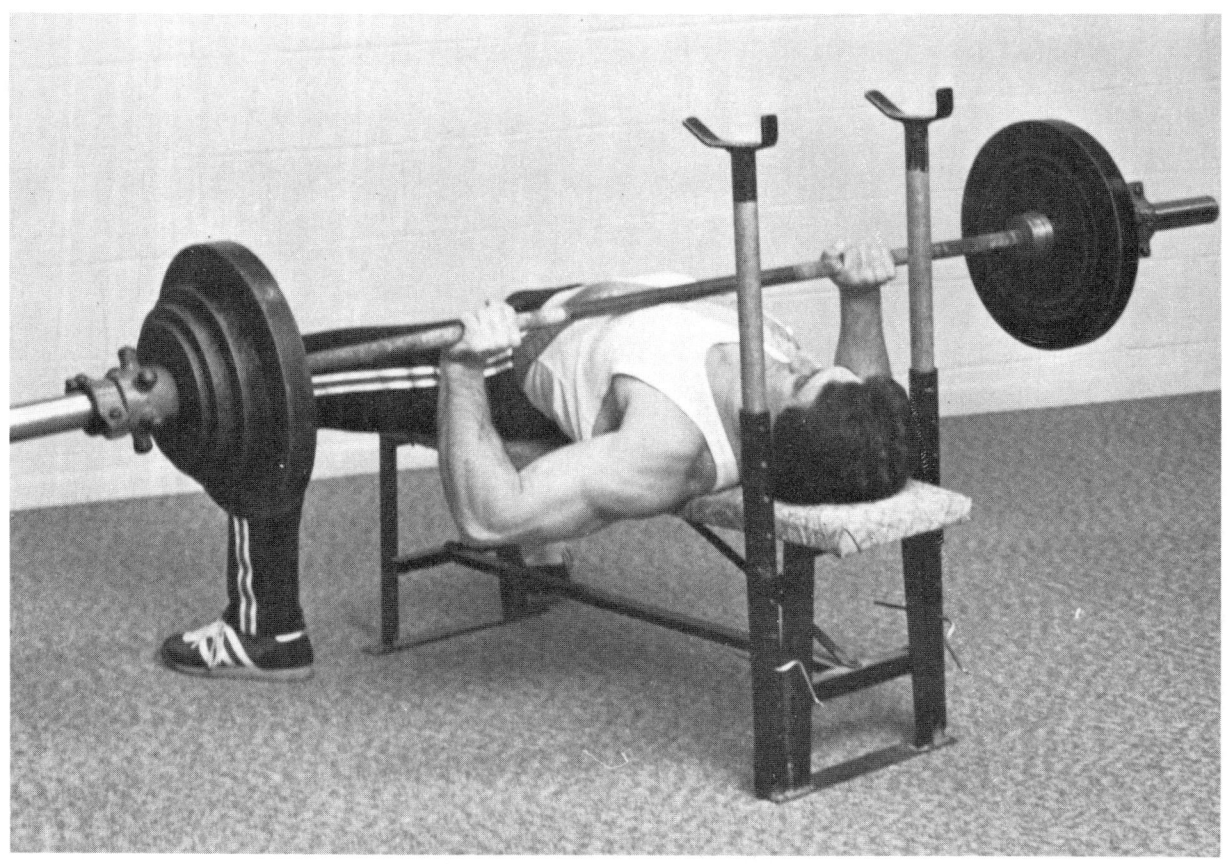

PROPER PERFORMANCE OF THE BENCH PRESS, as shown in the illustrations on this and the next page, is important for building chest, shoulder, and arm muscles. The bench press is used extensively in athletic conditioning as well as in bodybuilding.

your chest at the base of the pectoral muscles, near where these big chest muscles end on the rib cage, above the abdomen. As soon as the barbell touches your chest, push it back up to straight arms. You can begin to exhale as your arms straighten. Then inhale quickly and repeat for a total of eight presses.

In your first workout, experiment to determine how much weight you will need so that the final three repetitions (reps) to try. If it feels ridiculously light, try heavier weights until eight reps is no longer easy to complete. In subsequent workouts, take the same weight, but when it seems easy to complete eight reps, do one or two more. Also, add a second set, either with the same weight for approximately the same number of reps or with a few pounds more for a total of four to six reps.

When it becomes fairly easy to complete twelve reps with the starting weight, increase the poundage enough to restrict yourself to a comfortable eight reps again. Continue to add sets as well, either using the same weight or increasing the weight and decreasing the repetitions with each set. For example, suppose you start by doing eight reps with 50 pounds and

which can happen if you tackle a heavy weight without first doing easy work to get blood into the exercising muscles. For example, as you become more advanced, you might bench press 120 pounds eight to ten reps as a warm-up and then do three sets of eight with 150. Or do 120 × 8, 140 × 8, 150 × 6, and 160 × 4 if you are

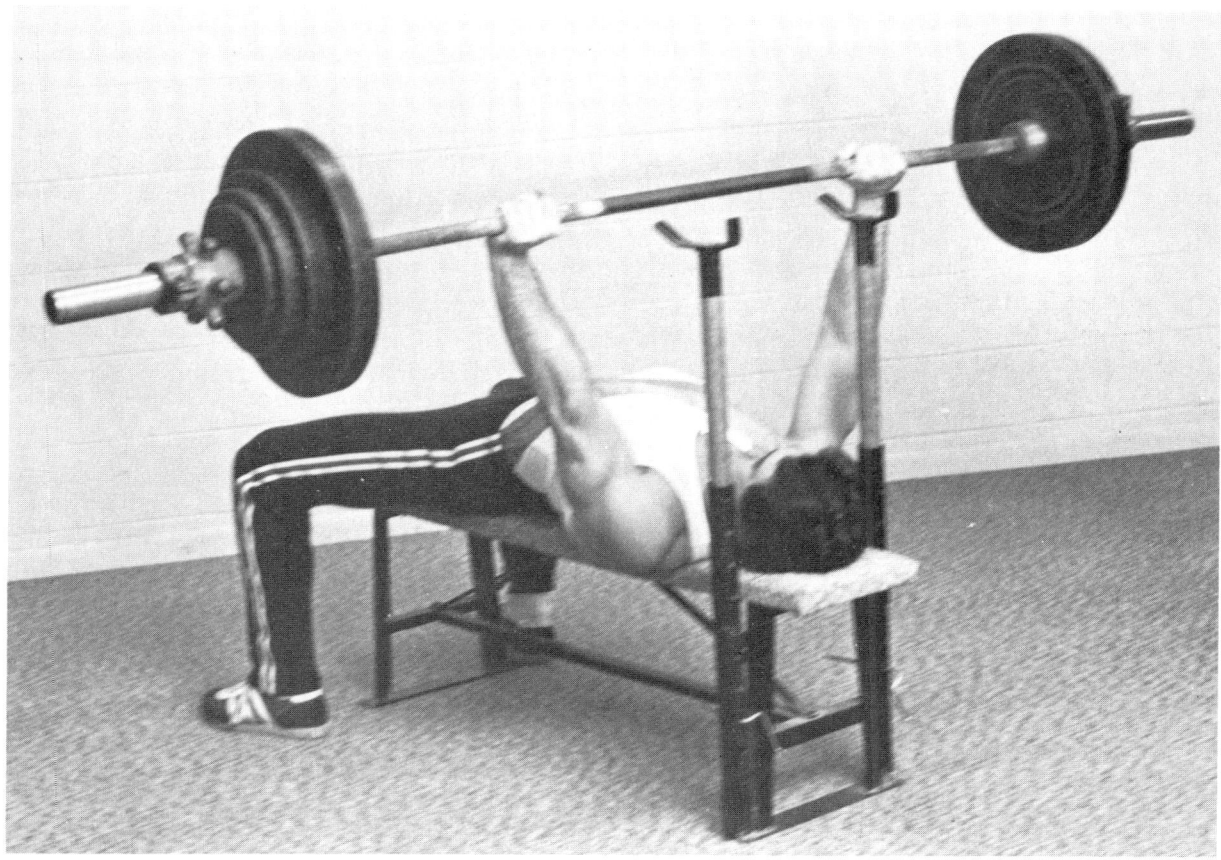

add sets and reps until you are doing 50 × 12 and 70 × 8 + 8 (two sets of eight). You then should be able to move up to start with 60 pounds for eight, followed by 75 pounds for two sets of five or six sets.

When you become strong enough to do eight reps with weights in the 150- to 200-pound range, you definitely should start with a deliberately light warm-up set, using a weight that is quite easy to handle for about eight reps. This will minimize any likelihood of muscle or tendon strain,

as interested in building strength as in bodybuilding effect.

Advanced Routines

As your strength and physical condition improve, additional bodybuilding effect can be obtained by working up with the weight for several sets and then finishing off with twelve to fifteen reps using a light weight. For example, if you were starting with 135 pounds, the weight of an Olympic-type barbell with a pair of 45-

pound plates, you would do eight reps to warm up and then 155 × 8, 170 × 6, 185 × 4, and 200 × 2. To finish off, you would drop back to 135 again and do as many as possible.

This approach is used by champion bodybuilders who seek great strength as well as muscular development. Franco Columbu, Mr. Olympia titlist, enjoys a workout in which he works up to more than 400 pounds in bench presses and then drops down to what would be a "light" weight for him, perhaps 225 pounds, for twelve or fifteen reps. Other champions will do a couple of warm-up sets with 135 and 225 pounds, eight to fifteen reps each, and then perform several sets with 315 pounds, striving to get six to ten reps in each set. Note the 90-pound increments. These very advanced men add a pair of 45-pound plates to the bar with each set!

Incidentally, many advanced bodybuilders stop just short of completely straightening their arms in the bench press in order to maintain continuous tension on the muscles being exercised. Others do lock their arms at the top of each press, but only momentarily, for the same reason.

You must use good judgment in determining how many repetitions you can complete with a given weight. The importance of having one or two training partners as "spotters," standing by to assist you if you can't complete a lift, can't be overemphasized. Bodybuilding is a relatively safe activity by comparison with most sports, but it literally is possible to be killed by a heavy barbell if you should fail with a heavy bench press while exercising alone.

Bench Press Benefits

The bench press usually is classified as a chest-building exercise because it devel-ops the size and strength of the pectoral muscles that cover the upper chest. It is also one of the best arm and shoulder exercises, especially for the front part of the shoulder (deltoid) muscles and the back part of the upper arm (triceps), the largest muscle mass of the arm. In addition, a person who gets the proper feel of doing bench presses will notice some response in the latissimus muscles that provide width to the back, since some tension in these "lats" helps support the upper arms at the start of the push from the chest (this is a tensing of the lats, not a true activation of these muscles, which work to pull the arms down and back). Because so many big muscles are involved in an exercise in which heavy weights can be used, the bench press is generally considered the best single upper-body exercise.

THE SQUAT

The second exercise that has been a key to the development of great strength and muscle size is the squat. Ideally, you should use squat stands, where you can place a light barbell or the empty bar ready for loading to the weight that will give your legs a suitable workout. If you don't have squat stands, you will need a couple of strong training partners to lift the barbell to your shoulders, for if you are dedicated in your training, you will soon be squatting with weights that one person will not be able to place there without strain.

To do the squat, place your hands fairly wide apart on the bar, with an overhand grip, as it rests on stands, and duck under it so that your head is centered as you come up. Rest the barbell across the back of your shoulders, below the prominent vertebra where your neck joins your upper back. You may want to wrap a towel around the center of the bar for comfort's sake. Lift the barbell off the supports by straightening your legs, and then step back so that you are clear of the supports. Keep your back flat and chest high, and lower your body smoothly by bending your knees until you are at a point where your thighs are approximately parallel with the floor. Rise immediately. Take a deep breath, high in your chest, before squatting and exhale as your legs are straightening the last few inches. Continue for eight reps, and then replace the barbell on the squat stands.

It is especially important not to permit your back to round as you do squats, and one way to determine the low position is to stop just above the point where you could not go any lower without rounding your low back.

Some exercise physiologists believe the supporting structures of the knees are overstretched to the point where the joints become vulnerable to injury if you do squats below the point where the tops of your thighs are approximately parallel with the floor (horizontal). Others disagree, and many instructors insist that the more completely the legs can be flexed, the more fully the thigh muscles will be developed. An excellent training effect can be obtained by going no lower than parallel, however, so if you are concerned about the possibility of overstretching your knees, stop when your thighs reach parallel. One way to determine when to rise is to stand with your back to a knee-high box or bench and squat until your buttocks touch it lightly.

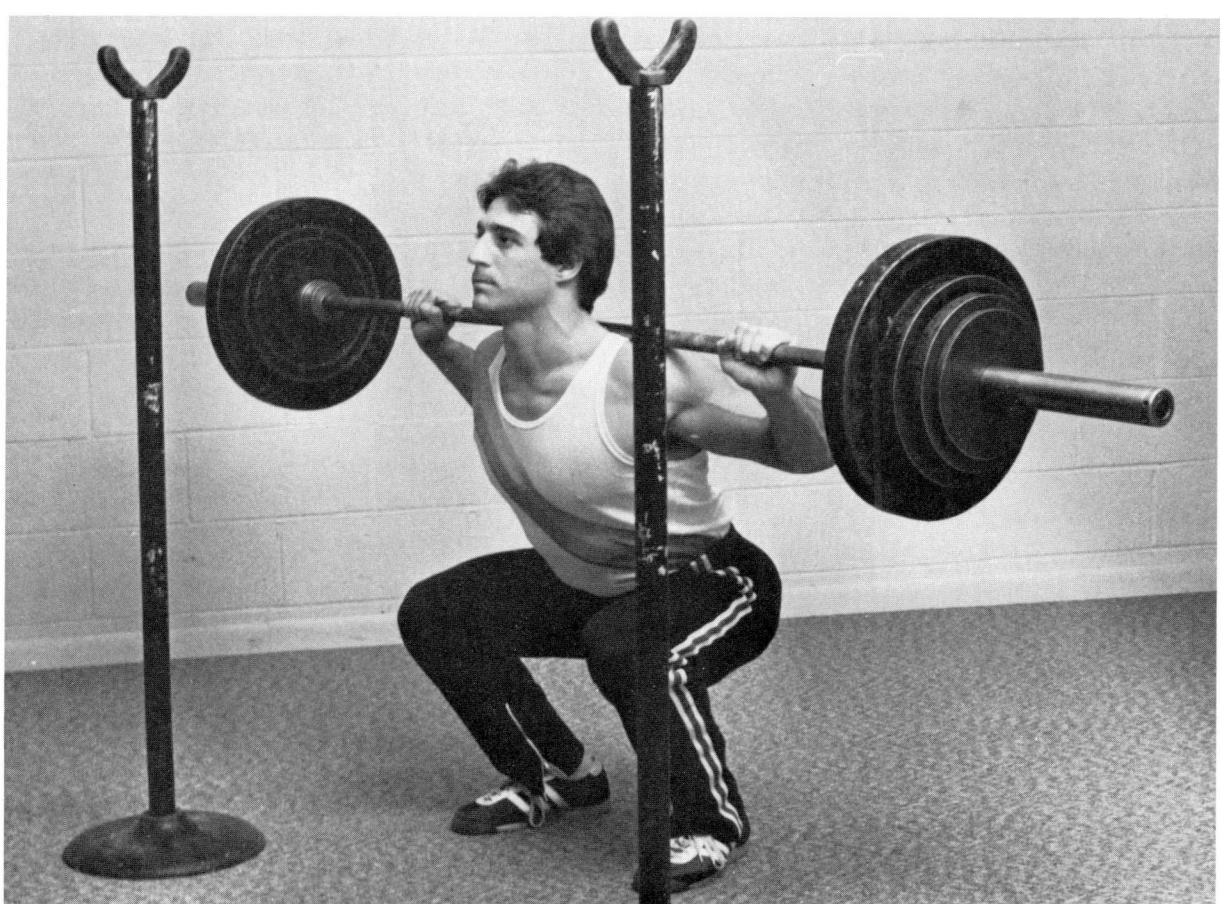

BOB CAPPIELLO shows correct position in the squat. Note that Bob, a former college soccer player, maintains a flat back and high chest and keeps his waist pulled in.

Concentrate on keeping your chest high and waist pulled in as you do squats. By doing this and keeping your back straight, you eliminate any tendency for the exercise to broaden your waistline by thickening the low back muscles toward the sides, above the buttocks. As with the arms in the bench press, many successful competitive bodybuilders stop just short of fully straightening their legs at the top of a squat. Others maintain tension on the frontal thigh muscles by making the lockout only momentary before starting down for the next repetition.

For most people, the best stance is with the feet placed about hip width and the toes pointing slightly outward. Feet should be kept flat on the floor so you can concentrate on forcing the leg muscles to work and on holding an erect position with the back flat. If you have a tendency for your heels to come off the floor at the lowest point of your squat, place a one-inch- or two-inch-thick board under your heels. You probably will not need to do this unless you intend to squat well below parallel. Also, the fact that you must keep your back flat does not mean that you should not incline your torso forward from the hips. You will need to lean forward somewhat, with a straight back, to maintain your balance.

Develop a Routine

Squats should be done much as bench presses are, starting with a relatively light warm-up set of eight or ten reps and then moving up to a weight that is challenging for the last two or three of eight to ten reps. For strength, add a third set with still more weight, enough to limit you to four or five reps.

Continue to work with the same weights until you can do the first set easily for ten to twelve, the second set for eight to ten, and the third set for at least six. For example, suppose you could do 120 × 10, 150 × 8, and 160 × 6. You should then move up to 125 × 10, 160 × 5-8 and 170 × 3-5. This approach will build strength and size.

Another approach is to do 120 × 10 and then three sets of eight to ten with 150. When you can get ten reps with all three sets with 150, you may move up to 125 × 10 and three sets of at least six, trying for eight or more, with 160. When you can do three sets of ten with 160, increase the weight again.

Squats, like bench presses, are done most safely with one or two training partners standing by as spotters in case you have trouble getting up. If you are training alone, resist the temptation to try one more rep if there is the slightest doubt in your mind about completing it.

As in the bench press, it is possible to handle very heavy weights in the squat. It is not unusual for leading competitive bodybuilders to exercise with 300 to 400 pounds or more for ten reps in the squat. Many—especially men like Franco Columbu who enjoy the challenge of heavy weights—will handle 500 pounds or more. But when the aim is to develop muscular and shapely legs, it is more important to feel the muscles working while doing repetitions than to stress handling ever heavier weights.

DEEP BREATHING PULLOVER

Pullovers are done after squats to take advantage of the need for repayment of oxygen debt by deep breathing and to give your body some rest from exercises requiring great energy expenditure. The recommended approach is to do a set of squats followed by a set of pullovers, so that the two exercises actually are done alternately rather than sets of one followed by sets of the other.

Remember, the basic eight exercises we

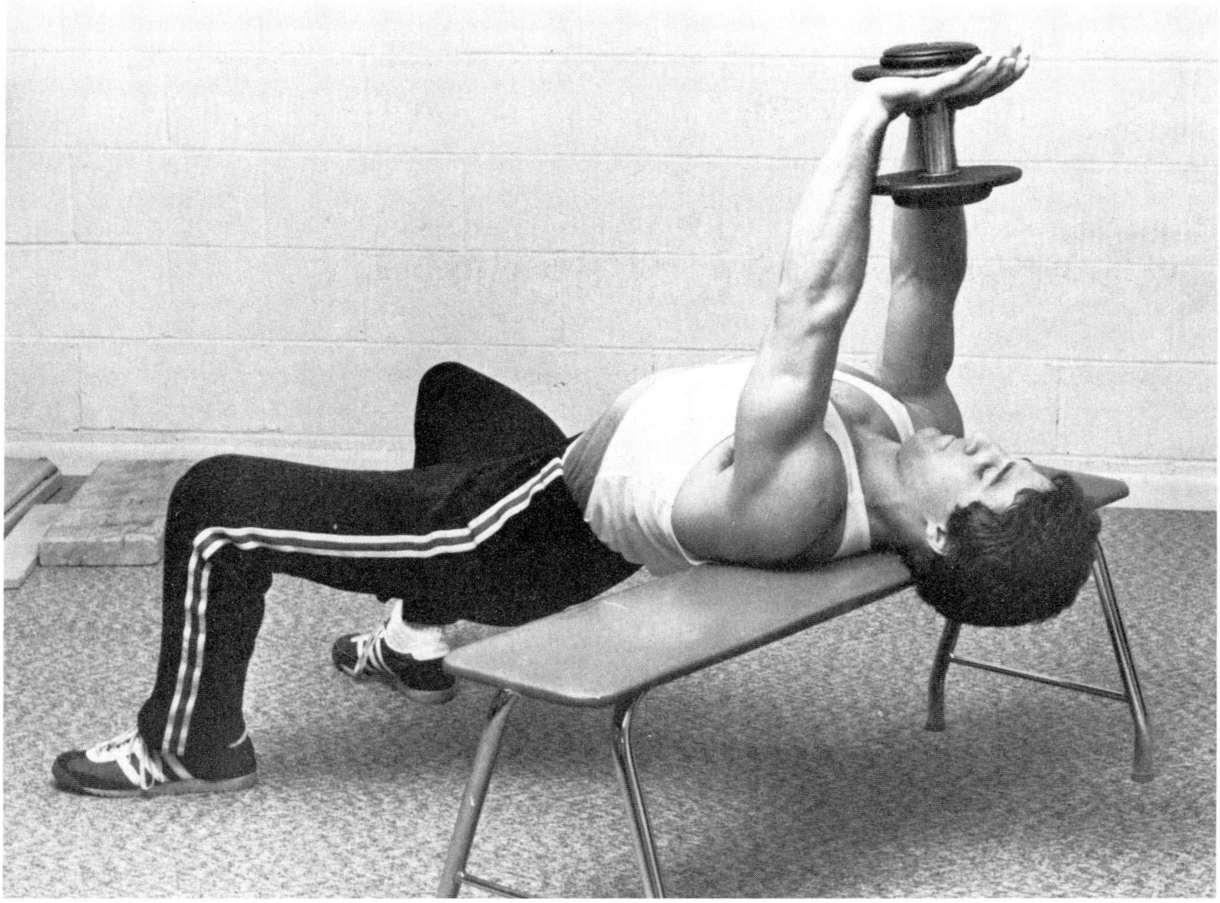

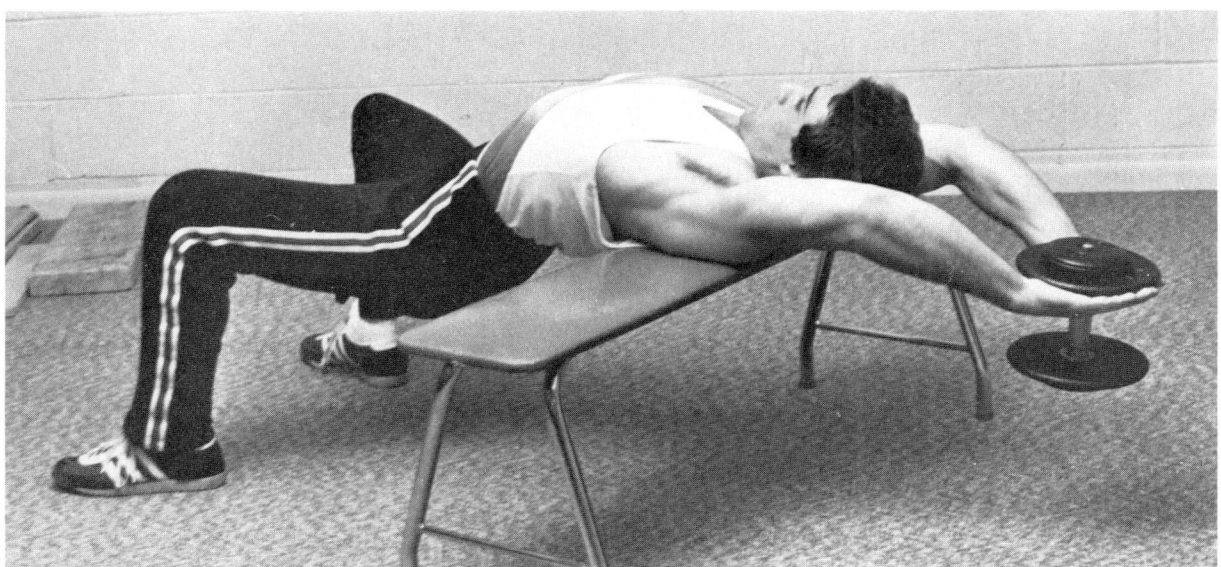

THE PULLOVER can be done with any compact, relatively light weight. The photos show the exercise with a single dumbbell. As the pictures show, the aim of the exercise is to stretch the chest and enlarge the rib cage.

are starting with call for no other equipment than a barbell, bench, and squat stands. Since any form of weight can be held in the hands to do pullovers, here is how to do them with a barbell.

Use a very light weight; the weight of the bar and collars is enough to start with. Grasp the bar with a narrow overhand grip—narrow enough so the tips of your thumbs touch when extended toward each other along the bar. Lie on your exercise bench (or the floor) with your head at the end, away from the pressing supports, and hold the bar straight up over your chest. Keeping your arms rigid (you may unlock your elbows slightly if it feels more comfortable to do so), lower the bar in an arc behind your head. Begin to inhale as you lower the bar. Time your inhalation so your lungs are full just before the bar reaches a fully-stretched position, as far down as you can lower it without hurting your shoulders. Immediately pull the bar back over to the starting point above your chest, exhaling as you raise it. Continue for a total of ten to twelve reps.

Instead of using a barbell, you may prefer to use a dumbbell handle or a piece of pipe about 14 inches long with one or two barbell plates in the center, held there by placing your hands against the plates on either side. Also, many leading bodybuilders do pullovers across a bench instead of lying on it. In this technique only the rib cage is supported, thus providing more stretch.

The pullover develops chest muscles and the latissimus muscles of the upper back; the primary aim is, however, to s-t-r-e-t-c-h the chest and expand the rib cage. So concentrate on stretching and full inhalation, only adding small amounts of weight when you feel you aren't getting enough stretch from the amount you're using.

ROWING EXERCISE

To develop the upper back, especially the big latissimus dorsi muscles (lats) that run from under the arms to the waist and impart a V-shape when developed, the best basic exercise is the rowing movement. To do it, grasp a barbell with an overhand grip, hands about shoulder-width apart, bend forward from the hips, keeping your back flat and horizontal,

WHEN DOING THE ROWING exercise for the latissimus muscles, the barbell should be pulled toward the waist, not straight up.

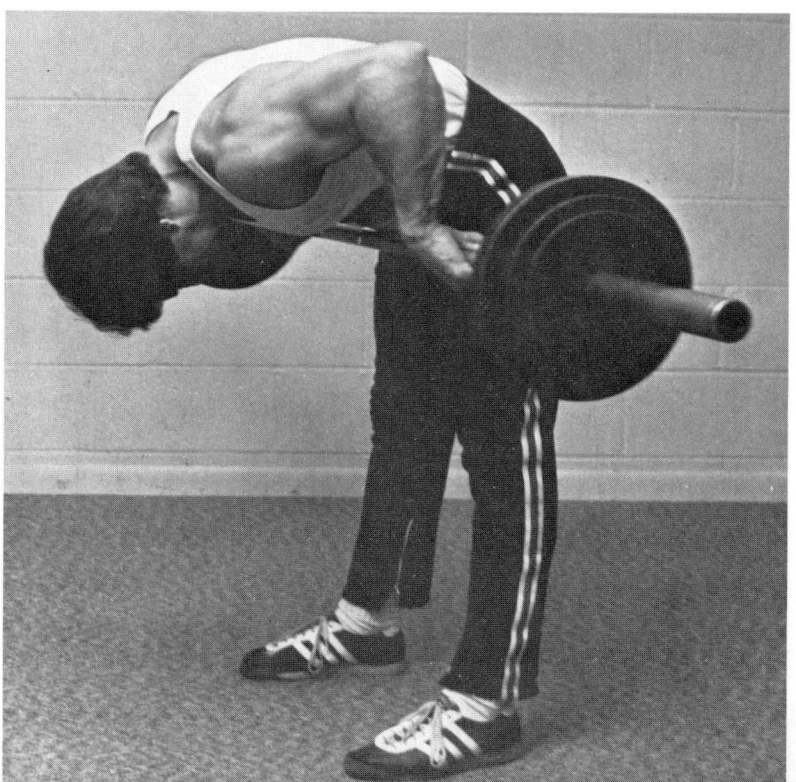

and pull the barbell up to touch your abdomen below your chest. The barbell should start from a hanging position directly below your shoulders, not touching the floor. You may bend your knees slightly for comfort to take the strain off your back and the backs of your legs.

Begin this exercise with a weight that permits about eight reps per set and increase the resistance five to ten pounds whenever it becomes easy to complete three sets of ten to twelve reps.

When doing the rowing exercise, don't just pull the weight up to touch your abdomen. If you do, you probably will overemphasize arm exercise to the neglect of the back muscles you are trying to develop. Instead, try to tense and contract your back muscles, and strive for the feeling that your back is working; your arms just go along for the ride to finish the motion. A good starting weight is

about 30 to 50 pounds, and when you can do three sets of ten with 100 pounds, you're getting pretty strong. Champion bodybuilders use 150 to 200 pounds and more.

THE CURL

The barbell curl is the basic biceps builder and it's done like this: grasp the barbell with an underhand grip, palms away from you, thumbs pointing outward, and hands spaced about shoulder-width apart. Stand erect with your arms hanging at your sides, the barbell resting across your upper thighs. Then flex your arms, keeping your elbows at your sides, so the barbell travels in an arc from your thighs to your upper chest.

Concentrate on contracting the biceps muscles while curling. Tense them deliberately as though you were "showing your muscle," and again let the weight go

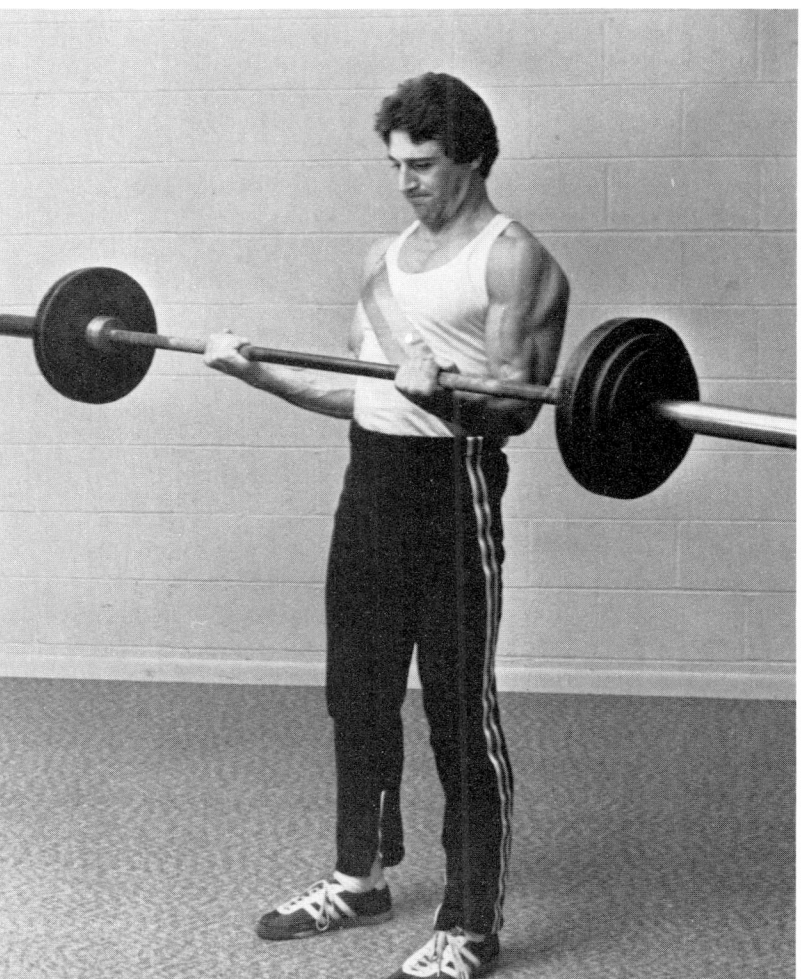

IN THE CURL the arm muscles are strenuously exercised, as the picture shows better than words can describe. This halfway position in the exercise is the most difficult point due to the leverage involved.

along for the ride. Try not to swing the weight up. Make the arm muscles do the work. Advanced bodybuilders handle heavy weights and get extra reps by "cheating"—swinging the weight with body motion to get it moving—but the ones who get the best results with a cheating motion are those who keep it to a minimum and still focus the work on their biceps.

How much weight should you use in the curl? Thirty to 50 pounds is enough for a beginner. Eighty to 100 pounds in good form takes a lot of strength, done for three sets of ten. Many advanced bodybuilding champions can do curls with 135 to 150 pounds without much cheating. A few men have been able to do single curls in good form with weights approximately equal to their body weights, and even heavier weights have been handled in looser style.

Incidentally, lower the weight—don't let it drop—when bodybuilding. The low-

ering motion also helps build muscle. This is especially important in an exercise that is focused on relatively small muscles, as is the curl. The biceps muscle lumps up impressively when the arm is flexed, but it is a relatively small muscle by comparison with the triceps, the pectorals of the chest, or the big quadriceps of the thighs.

Barbell curls should be begun with a weight that will permit eight reps, and you should add sets to three and reps to twelve. The add 5 to 10 pounds and start over at three sets of eight, again attempting to work up to twelve before adding weight.

THE RISE-ON-TOES

To develop the calf muscles of the lower leg from the back of the knee to the heel, you must contract and stretch them fully, working against substantial resistance. There are many pieces of apparatus that make it possible to do this exercise conve-

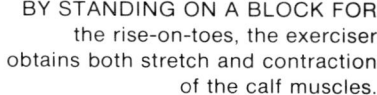

BY STANDING ON A BLOCK FOR
the rise-on-toes, the exerciser
obtains both stretch and contraction
of the calf muscles.

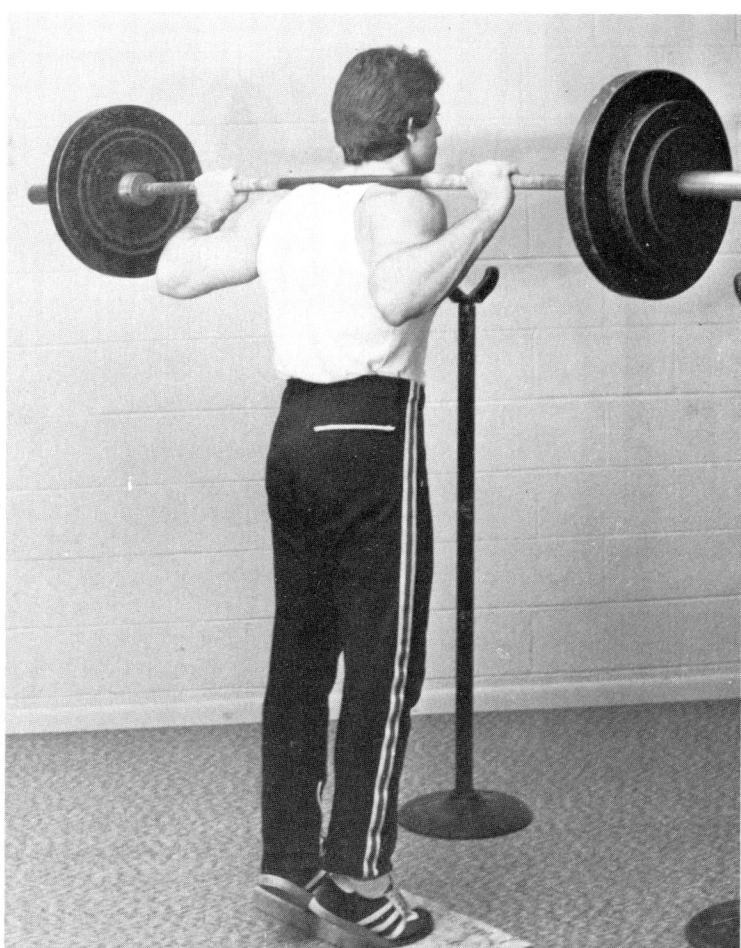

niently, but it can be done with no more equipment than a barbell and a small section of wood one to two inches thick.

Hold the barbell across your shoulders (squat stands provide a convenient means of shouldering it), and stand with your toes and the balls of your feet elevated on the one- to two-inch thick block of wood. Then alternately rise as high as possible on your toes and lower your heels to full stretch, touching them to the floor below the block. Do five to ten reps with your toes pointed straight ahead, five to ten with toes pointed outward, and five to ten with your toes pointed inward to fully work the calf muscles (primarily the gastrocnemius, the upper area).

Select an amount of weight that causes you to feel the muscle working. The calf muscles are dense and strong because they are constantly activated as you walk, but if it is difficult to complete fifteen to thirty reps with 100 pounds, then 100 pounds is enough weight. Many advanced bodybuilders do the exercise with 200 pounds and more, but this is because they work calf muscles so much that they need a lot of resistance to feel any effect from the exercise.

THE SIT-UP

Many variations of sit-ups are touted by different instructors and best-built-man contest winners, and all of them will work the abdominal muscles if they are done properly, vigorously, and regularly. An effective method that is easily learned is as follows:

Lie supine and have your feet held down by a training partner or tuck them under an object that will hold them down. Bend your knees. Clasp your hands behind your head. Take a deep breath and deliberately exhale. As you exhale, pull your abdomen in, cock your hips up and your head forward so your chin approaches your chest. Then sit up, touch-

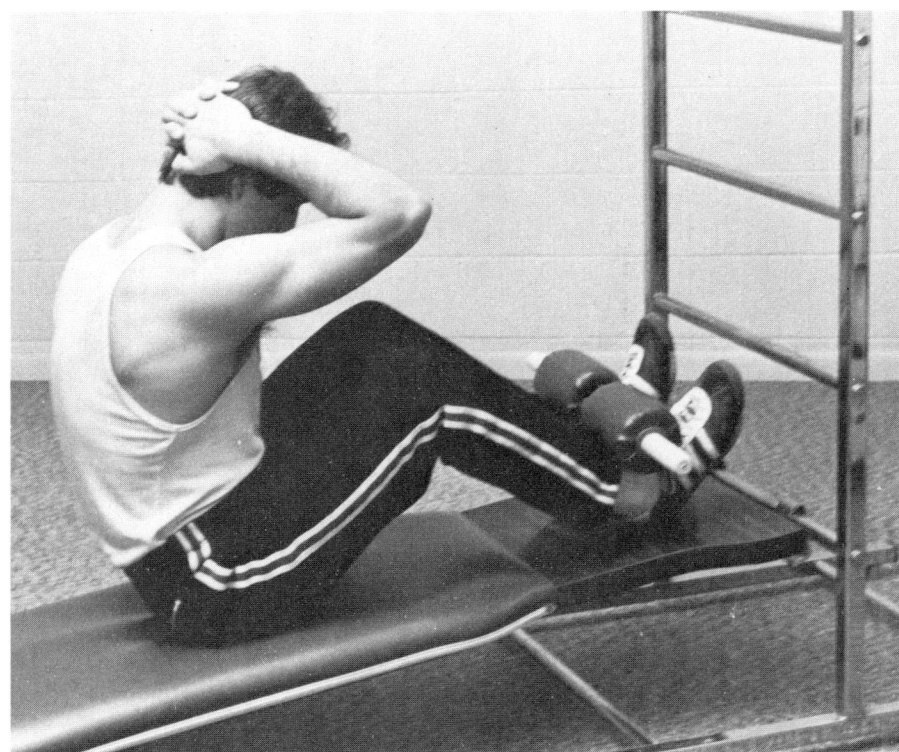

SIT-UPS should be done with knees bent. A slanted abdominal board adds to the difficulty of the exercise.

ing your elbows to your knees. Lower yourself to the starting position and repeat.

With each repetition, consciously exhale and pull your abdomen in deliberately as you sit up. Don't rush the exercise. Take enough time with each sit-up to feel the muscles tighten as you make the effort. Do at least ten reps and try for twenty. If you can only do ten or less, add a set with each workout until you are doing three sets for a total of about thirty sit-ups, counting all the reps of the three sets.

Most leading competitive bodybuilders —men whose abdominal muscles stand out like bricks in a wall—do fifty or more reps in abdominal exercises, though some capable instructors believe the abdominal muscles should be worked hard against resistance for no more repetitions than any other muscle. Both approaches seem to produce results, providing the person doing the exercises also watches his diet carefully, eliminating or reducing to a minimum fattening foods that are high in carbohydrates.

A good goal is to work up to fifty sit-

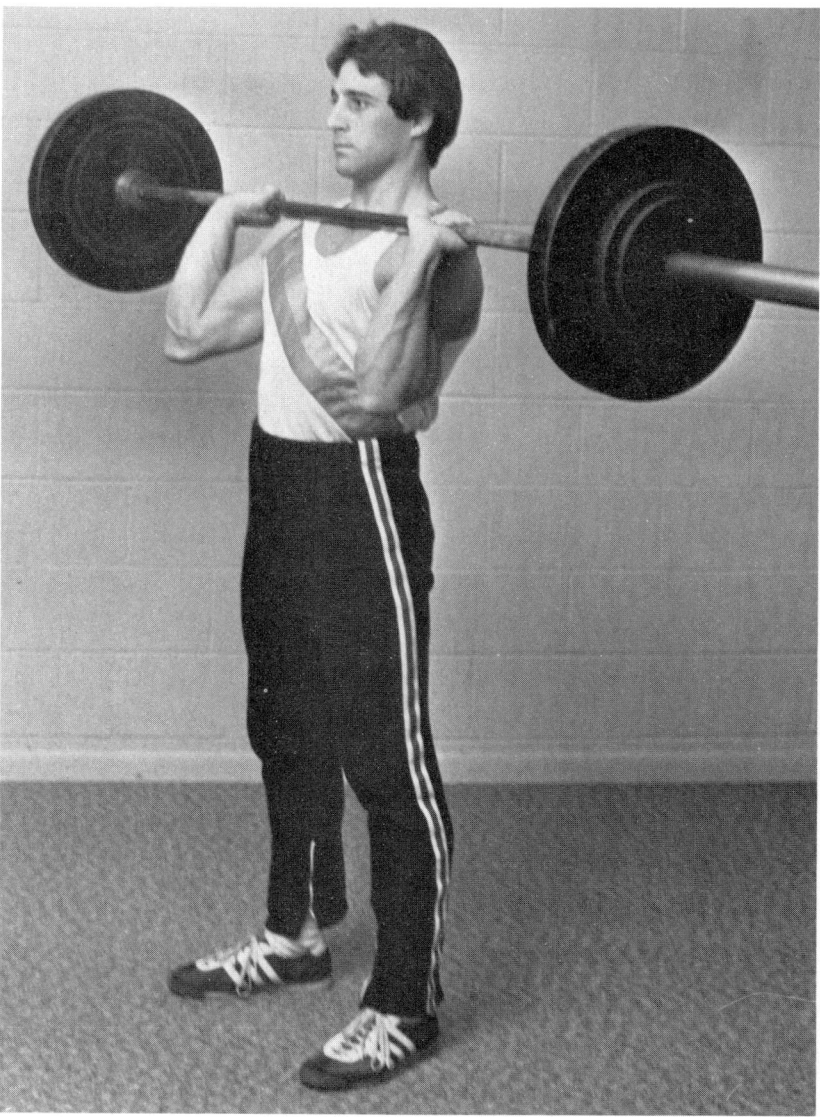

THE BARBELL PRESS, as shown here and on page 33, is one of the best shoulder-developing exercises.

ups for one set. If your abdomen still seems to need more work, add a second set (do one set at the start of your workout and one near the end.) If your midsection is trim but not muscular, do the sit-ups with a 10-pound weight held behind your head. Remember, however, that if you want sharply defined abdominal muscles, you will have to control your diet as well as exercise.

BARBELL PRESS

The final exercise in this basic, eight-exercise program is the barbell press, either standing or seated. This exercise is done with an overhand grip, thumbs inward on the barbell, hand spaced two to four inches wider than shoulder-width. Begin by lifting the barbell to your chest with a clean motion, as follows:

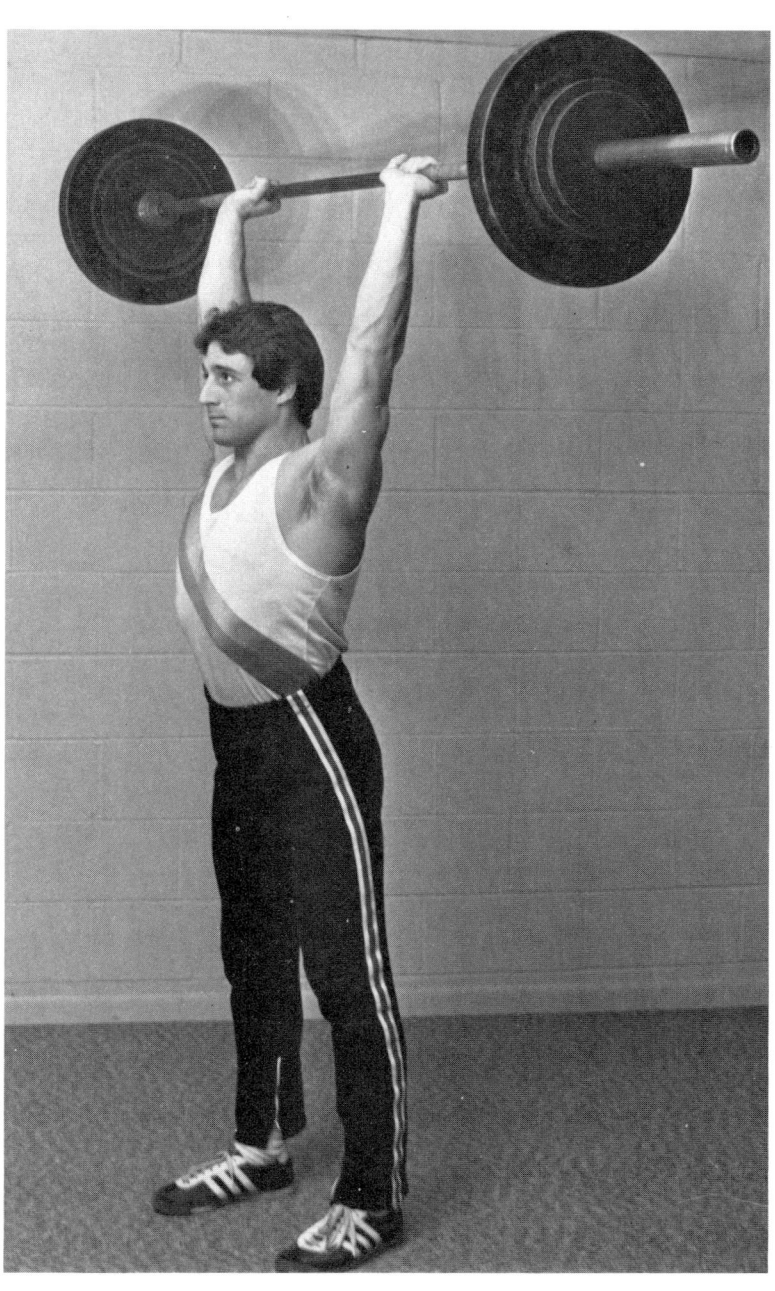

Stand close to the barbell so that the bar is over your insteps and your toes are projecting past it, feet about hip-width apart. Crouch and grasp the bar; then consciously flatten your back and lower your hips so that your hips are lower than your shoulders. With your arms hanging straight, begin to straighten your legs, which will raise the barbell off the floor. As the bar passes your knees, consciously bring it back toward your thighs and pull hard with your arms, continuing to straighten your legs and back (which should remain flat throughout). As the barbell passes your abdomen, continue to pull with your arms. The quickly turn your hands over and thrust your elbows down and forward to catch the barbell across your upper chest and the front of your shoulders.

With the weight at your chest, stand erect with legs straight, take a breath, and push the weight past your face, straight overhead to fully locked arms. Exhale as your arms straighten and, without hesitating, let the weight down to your chest smoothly, inhaling as it reaches your chest, and immediately push (press) it back overhead again. Experiment to find a weight you can press eight times with difficulty, but less than an all-out effort. Add sets to three and try to add repetitions with each workout until you can do three sets of ten to twelve. Then add five or ten pounds and begin the progression again at eight reps.

The press is one of the best exercises for the deltoid muscles that cap the shoulders, and it also works the triceps as you straighten your arms. Many people who have good natural leverage for bodybuilding exercises also are good pressers, both on the bench and overhead. A good goal is to do three sets of eight to ten reps with 100 pounds on the barbell, but many topflight bodybuilders can do this exercise with 200 pounds or more.

SHAPING EXERCISES

All bodybuilding exercises, including the eight muscle-building movements described previously, improve the shape of the body. But additional shaping exercises also should be included in a complete routine. The eight basic movements, done with reasonably heavy weights on a barbell, were given in a sequence that places the two major muscle-building, energy-requiring exercises first, then proceeds through key exercises for every part of the body. The shaping exercises to be described next should be included in the workout after the key heavy moves, so that you are "flushing" the area with blood by adding work for the same area that has been activated by the preceding exercise.

You can also "superset" the exercises. That is, you can do two exercises for the same body part alternately. For example, you might superset bench presses and the flying exercise (below) for the pectorals. Or you might superset exercises for antagonistic muscles, such as the curl for the biceps (arm flexors) and a triceps extension (for the extensors).

THE FLYING EXERCISE

This exercise, which focuses on the pectoral muscles of the chest, is done lying supine on a bench, using two dumbbells. Holding a dumbbell in each hand directly over your chest as you lie supine, turn your palms inward (toward each other) and unlock your elbows, keeping your arms bent throughout the exercise. Start by lowering the dumbbells to your sides, increasing the bend somewhat if necessary to get a full stretch of your chest muscles without straining your arms and shoulders. Inhale as you lower the weights to your sides, and then immediately try consciously to contract your chest muscles in order to pull the dumb-

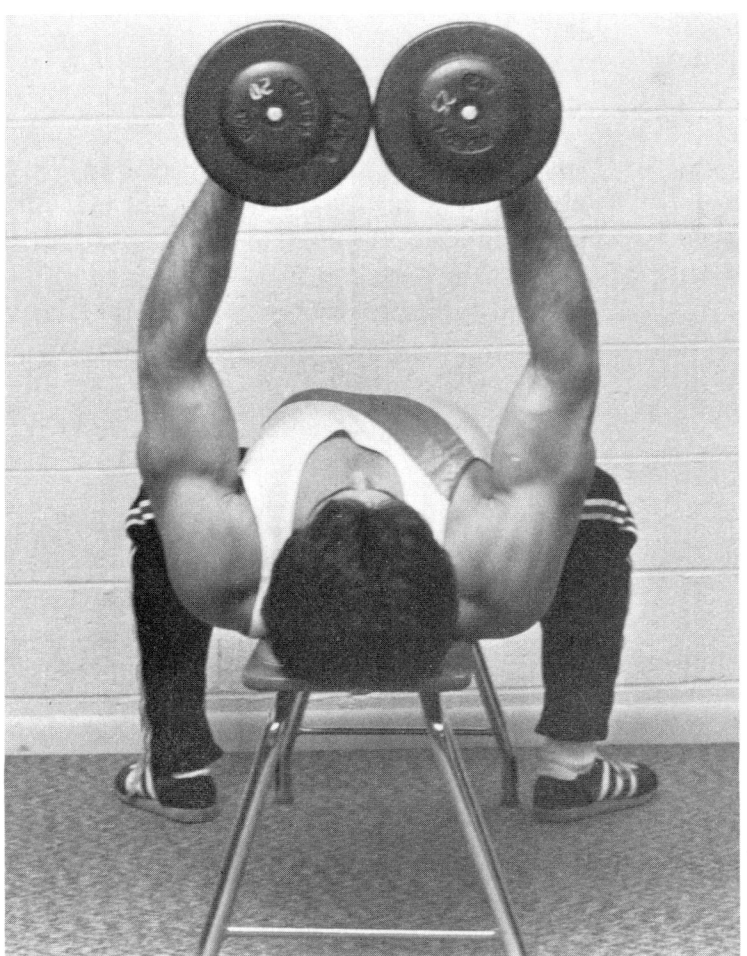

THE "FLYING" EXERCISE stretches and contracts the pectoral muscles of the chest, as the pictures show. Bending the elbows reduces strain on the joints.

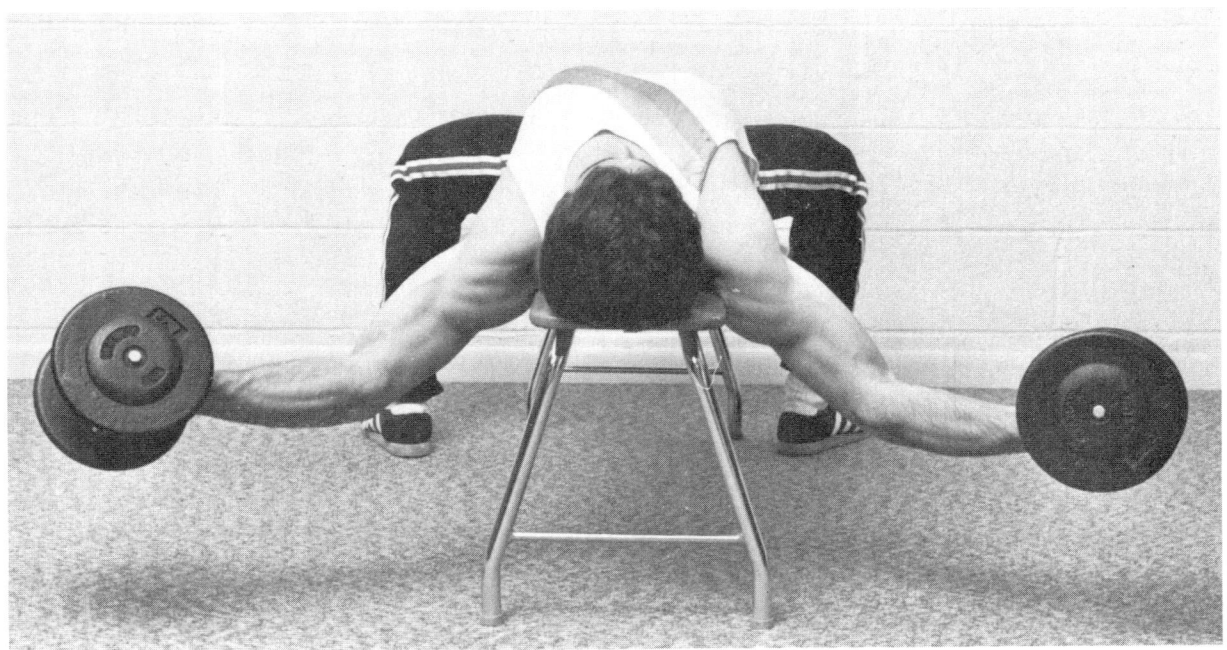

bells back together above your chest, exhaling. Continue for ten to twelve repetitions and add sets to three.

The flying exercise, using moderately weighted dumbbells, is a good one to superset with bench presses, doing a set of "flys" (often spelled "flyes" in bodybuilding magazines) after each set of bench presses. Or you might do three or more sets of bench presses followed by three or more sets of flys.

The flying exercise is called "flying" because the motion of the arms is like the action of a bird's wings, only inverted. The performance of the exercise varies a great deal from one individual to another, some keeping their arms bent but rigid, while others increase the bend so much as the weights are lowered that they almost are performing bench presses with dumb-

bells. The less the arms are bent, the greater the leverage against the muscles, so light dumbbells can be used effectively (dumbbells weighing from 5 pounds each for beginners to 20 or 30 pounds for advanced men). With more bending and straightening of the arms, more weight is needed to work the muscles thoroughly.

The important thing to remember is to bring the weights back up by contracting the pectoral muscles, not by working the arms and shoulders. I personally believe it is easier to focus the work on the pectorals if the weights are kept relatively light and the arms are held in a rigidly bent position, not changing the angle of bend as the weights are raised and lowered.

Franco Columbu, Mr. Universe and Mr. Olympia titlist, has found that he can get the proper feel of pectoral stretch and

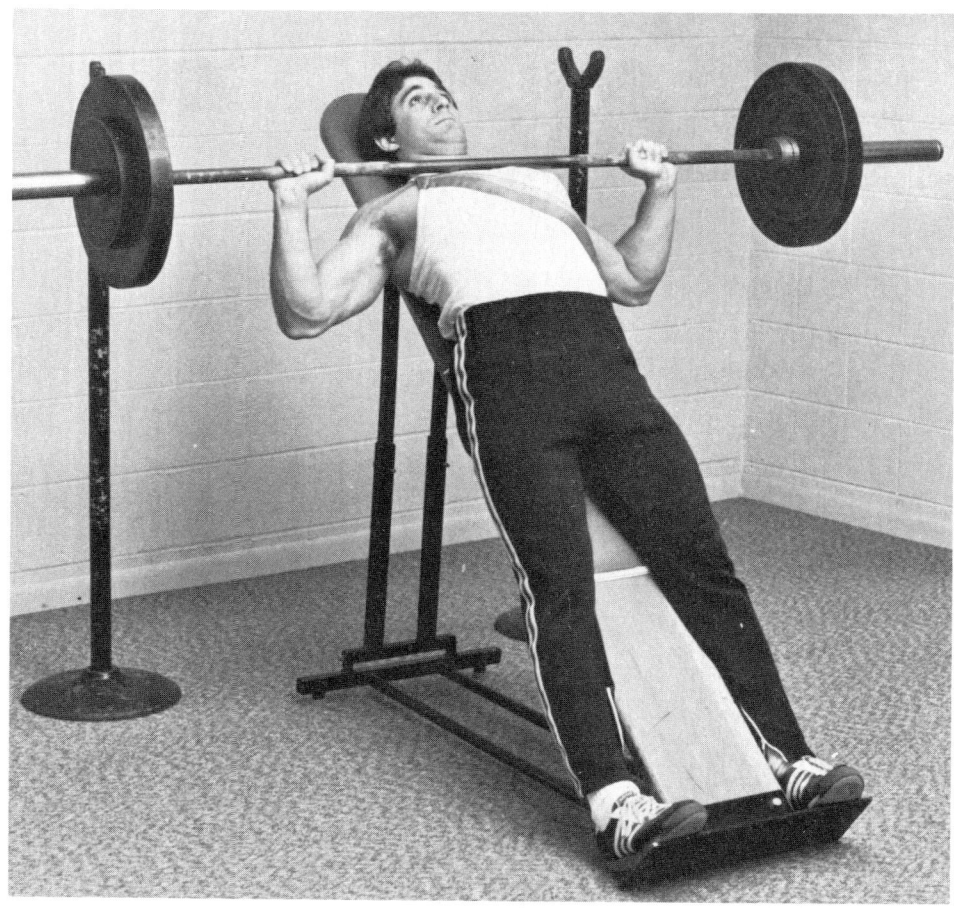

THE INCLINE PRESS (shown here and on the next page) can be done with a barbell or two dumbbells. Dumbbells are more effective for bodybuilding because they permit more downward stretch at the start.

contraction with considerable bend at the low position and almost straight arms with the dumbbells over his chest. Photos show his method in *Winning Bodybuilding*, a Contemporary Sports Books publication that I strongly commend to your attention, especially if you are thinking of entering competition.

In performing the flying exercise, you can direct the work to the upper part of the pectoral muscles by elevating the head-end of the bench two to six inches. You can direct the work to the lower part of the pectorals by elevating the foot-end of the bench.

THE INCLINE PRESS

Another of the best pectoral-developing exercises, one that ties in the anterior deltoids and also helps build the arms, is the incline press. Incline presses can be done with two dumbbells or a barbell, but they require a specially designed bench, tilted at about a 45-degree angle. A sturdy board, tilted at about the same angle and braced so it will not tip or slip, also will serve the purpose.

To do the exercise, hold a pair of dumbbells so that the handles point straight out from your ears, the inside of the dumbbells touching the outer part of

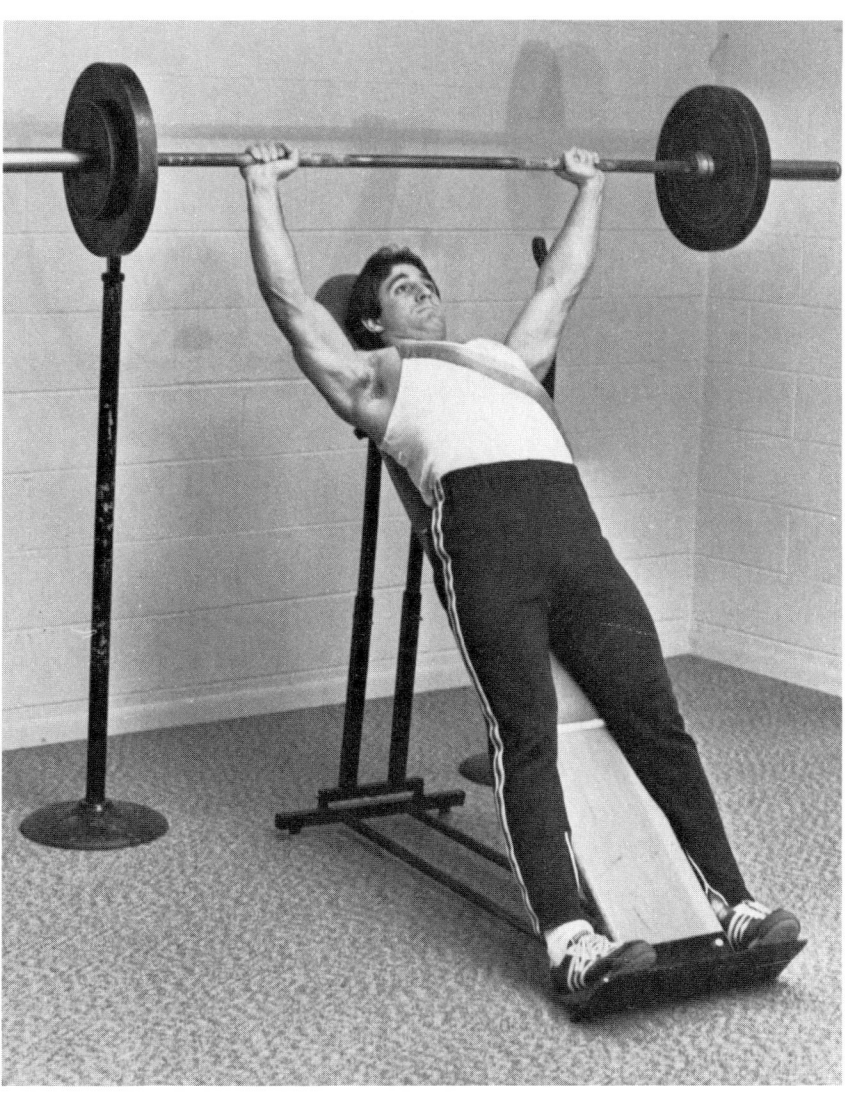

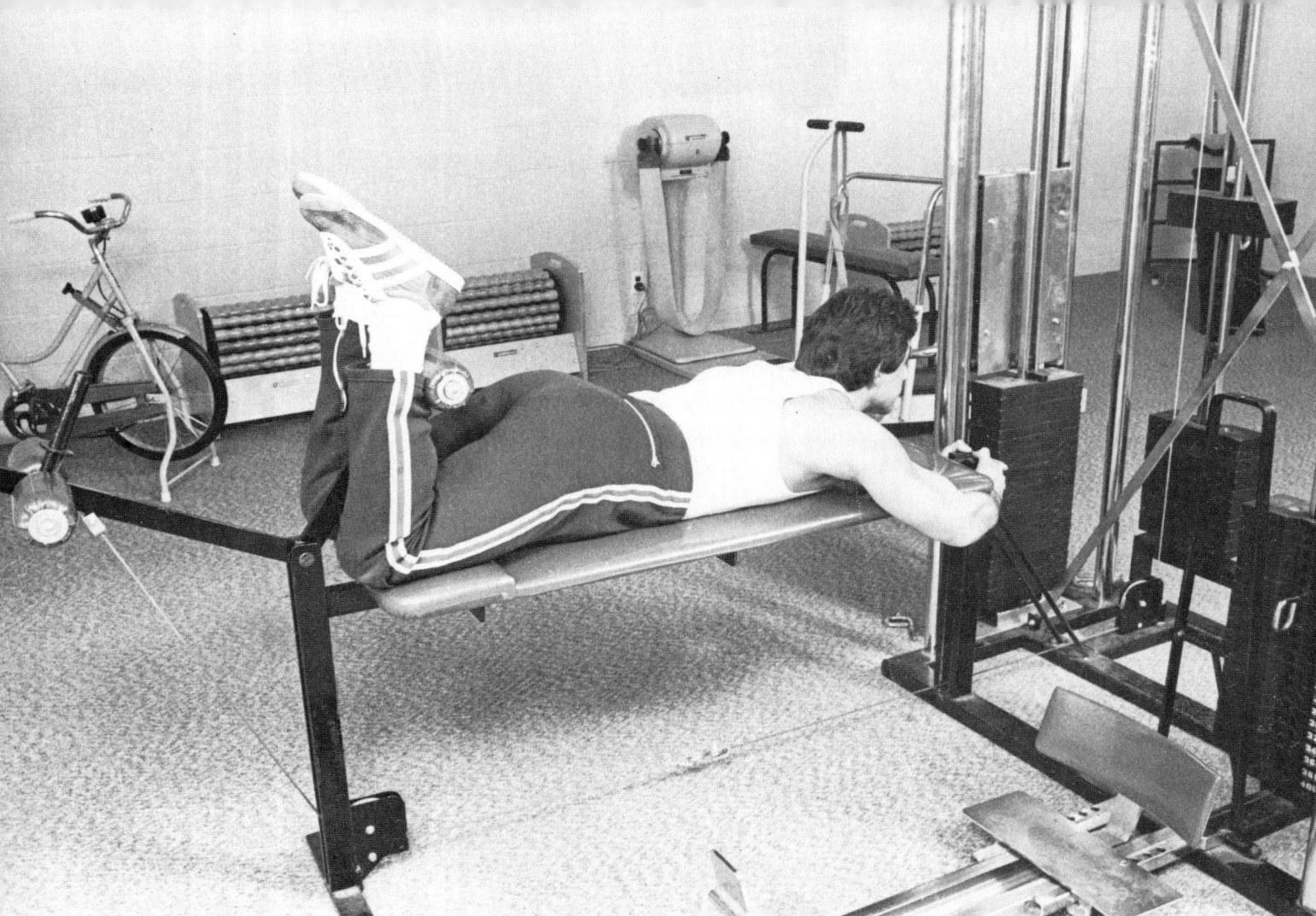

THE LEG CURL, the best direct exercise for the hamstrings (thigh biceps), is most conveniently performed on special apparatus, as shown. It can be done with dumbbells or a barbell attached to metal sandals, however, if no leg curl machine is available.

your shoulders. Lean against the bench, and press the dumbbells straight up eight to ten reps, three sets. The fact that you are leaning against an angled bench places the strain on the upper part of the pectoral muscles and results in a high-chested appearance.

The exercise can be done in the same way with a barbell, but dumbbells provide more stretch as you lower them to the sides of your shoulders and thus are more effective for bodybuilding.

THE LEG CURL

Squats are the main leg-developing exercise, but they mostly affect the muscles at the front and sides of the legs, having minimum effect on the biceps of the thighs (hamstrings), muscles that run up the backs of the legs from the knees to the buttocks. In order to work the thigh biceps directly, it is necessary to perform a leg-flexing exercise against resistance that is similar to the arm curling motion.

Ideally, the place to do leg curls is at a gym or health club, where special leg-curling apparatus is available. If you do not have access to a gym or club, however, you can do the exercise by obtaining metal sandals called "iron boots." These devices are designed so dumbbell bars can be attached, and you can perform the leg curl one leg at a time, standing with the non-exercising foot elevated on an object high enough so that the boot and dumbbell do not touch the floor.

Leg curls should be done from one to three sets of eight to ten repetitions. It's especially important to do this exercise if the back of your thigh is flat or poorly shaped.

LEG EXTENSIONS

An excellent exercise for the front of the thigh, to shape and define the muscles, is the leg extension. As with the leg curl, this exercise is best done on special apparatus available in gyms and health clubs, but it is another one that you can do in your home gym by using an iron boot with a dumbbell attached.

In this exercise, sit on a sturdy table with your thigh supported to the knee, the lower leg with weight attached hang- ing straight down. Then simply extend (straighten) the leg until it points straight out from the table. Do one to three sets of ten to twelve reps.

Incidentally, this exercise is a favorite of physical therapists. It can be used to rehabilitate an injured knee gradually, since you can begin with the lightest of weights and there is no stress on the knee due to the body's weight. Yet leg exten- sions strongly activate the muscles that straighten the leg and stabilize the knee.

Leg curls and extensions should be done after squats, not supersetted with them. These two exercises can be super- setted alternately with each other, how- ever, though most bodybuilders seem to prefer to finish all the sets of one before moving on to the other.

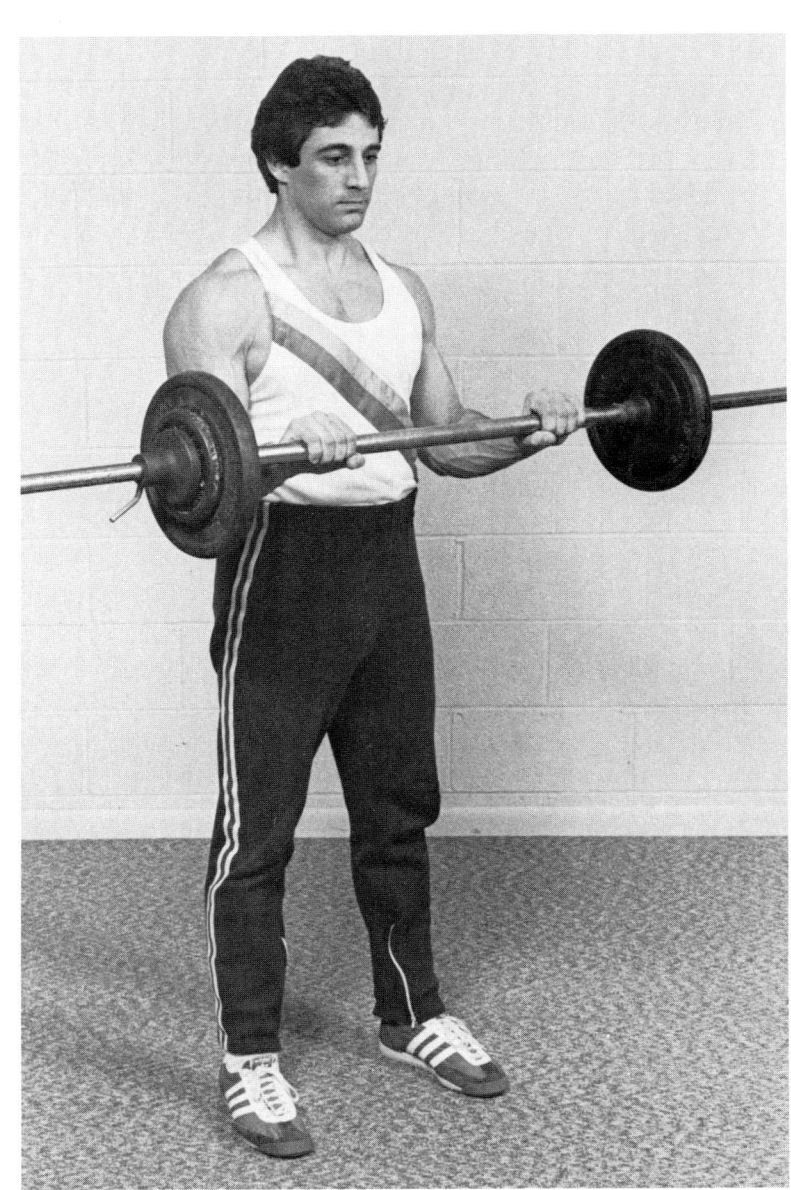

THE REVERSE CURL, with knuckles up, develops forearm muscles and strengthens the grip.

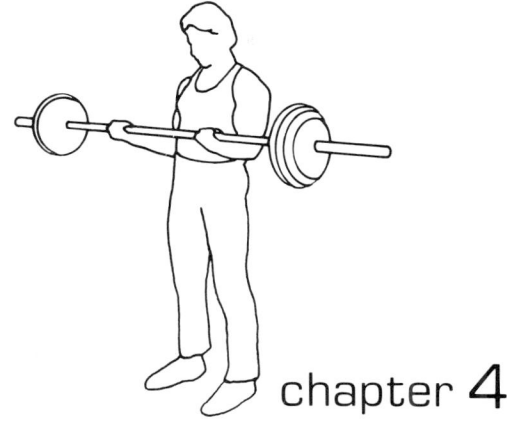

chapter **4**

ADDITIONAL EXERCISES

THE FRONT SQUAT

A variation on the regular squat exercise is to perform squats while holding a barbell across your upper chest and the front of your shoulders instead of on the back of your shoulders behind your neck. The leverage is much tougher when you hold the weight at your chest, and if you keep your body properly erect and your back flat, more work is placed on the thigh muscles close to the knees. Because of the leverage, it may be necessary to place a thicker board under your heels for the front squat than for the regular squat.

Steve Reeves, the Mr. America and Mr. Universe winner who went on to gain fame as a motion picture Hercules, was very conscious of the contrast between his wide shoulders and unusually narrow

hips. To accentuate this, he selected exercises that would develop his latissimus muscles and was careful to place minimal strain on his hips while exercising his legs. He did front squats with his heels elevated on a thick board, with feet only about six inches apart and pointed straight ahead, concentrating on holding himself very erect and attempting to focus the work on the lower part of his thighs. With this method, he was able to obtain a good workout for his thighs with relatively light weights. For a man of his size and strength, 150 pounds was "light," but he made the exercise effective by concentrating on correct performance.

Front squats should be done in sets of eight to twelve reps, or in higher repetitions (to fifteen) if additional leg work is needed.

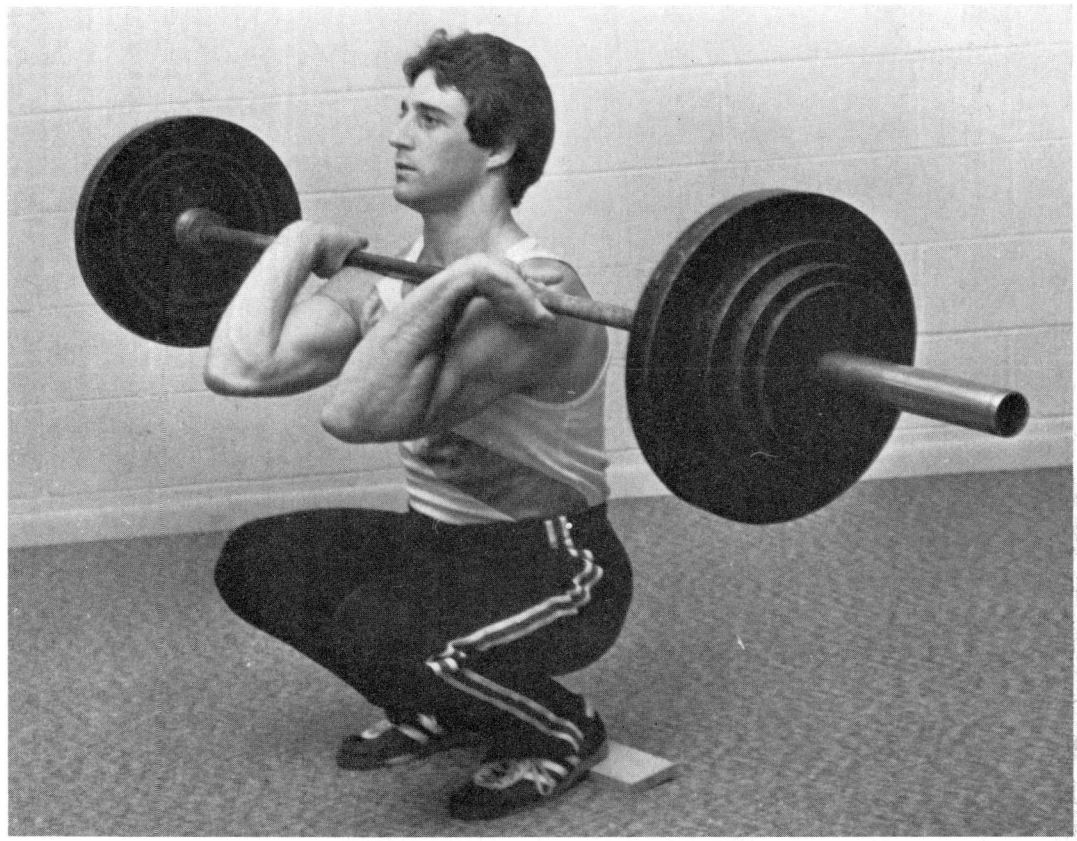

FRONT SQUATS are more difficult than regular squats because the leverage is less favorable. The exercise is especially effective for developing the lower part of the thighs.

THE BENT-ARM PULLOVER

The regular pullover is done with relatively light weights and is primarily a chest stretching exercise, but the bent-arm pullover is done with as much weight as can be used for eight to ten reps and is intended to build upper-body muscle. The exercise is done lying supine on a bench, some exercisers preferring to have their heads hanging over the end and others preferring to have their heads supported by the bench. The reason many prefer to have their heads hang over is that this places less restriction on the mobility of the shoulders.

While lying on the bench, reach back with arms bent and grasp a barbell placed close to the end of the bench. Grasp it with an overhand grip (in this case, over-hand will place your knuckles under the bar), thumbs inward, hands spaced six to ten inches apart. Keeping your elbows bent, pull the weight up past your head and face, and touch the bar to your chest. Lower and repeat for a total of eight to ten pullovers.

You should keep the barbell close to your face while performing bent-arm pullovers, but be careful not to use so much weight that you can't avoid contact. Contact with a barbell on any part of the face can be painful indeed!

This simple exercise especially builds the latissimus dorsi muscles of the upper back, the pectorals and serratus muscles of the chest, and the triceps of the arms. Some exotic devices have been developed for adding to the effectiveness of the bent-arm pullover, in particular the "Nautilus" and other similar machines utilizing cams. But excellent results can be achieved with no more equipment than a barbell and a bench.

An appropriate point at which to add bent-arm pullovers to our eight-exercise basic routine is right after the rowing motion. Thirty pounds is enough to experiment with at the start, but 100 pounds is within reach of most serious exercisers in time. Some strong body-builders use 150 to 200 pounds or more in this exercise. Back in the 1940s, Steve Stanko—who was first a weight lifting champion and later winner of Mr. America and Mr. Universe titles—used to perform a bent-arm pullover with well over 300 pounds. He then would bench press the weight, still using the less-than-shoulder-width grip that he employed for the pullovers!

CURL VARIATIONS

There are many variations of the basic curl with barbell, one of the very best being the curl with two dumbbells. Dumbbells are more difficult to exercise with than a barbell because you must control two independently moving objects rather than focus your attention on the single barbell. However, the fact that you must handle exactly the same amount with each arm provides a bodybuilding advantage. That is, you must do equal work with each arm rather than subconsciously take more of the strain on your better-coordinated side, as you can with a barbell.

Another advantage of curling with dumbbells is that you can rotate your wrists in a natural motion that permits the biceps to carry out their normal functions without hindrance. When curling

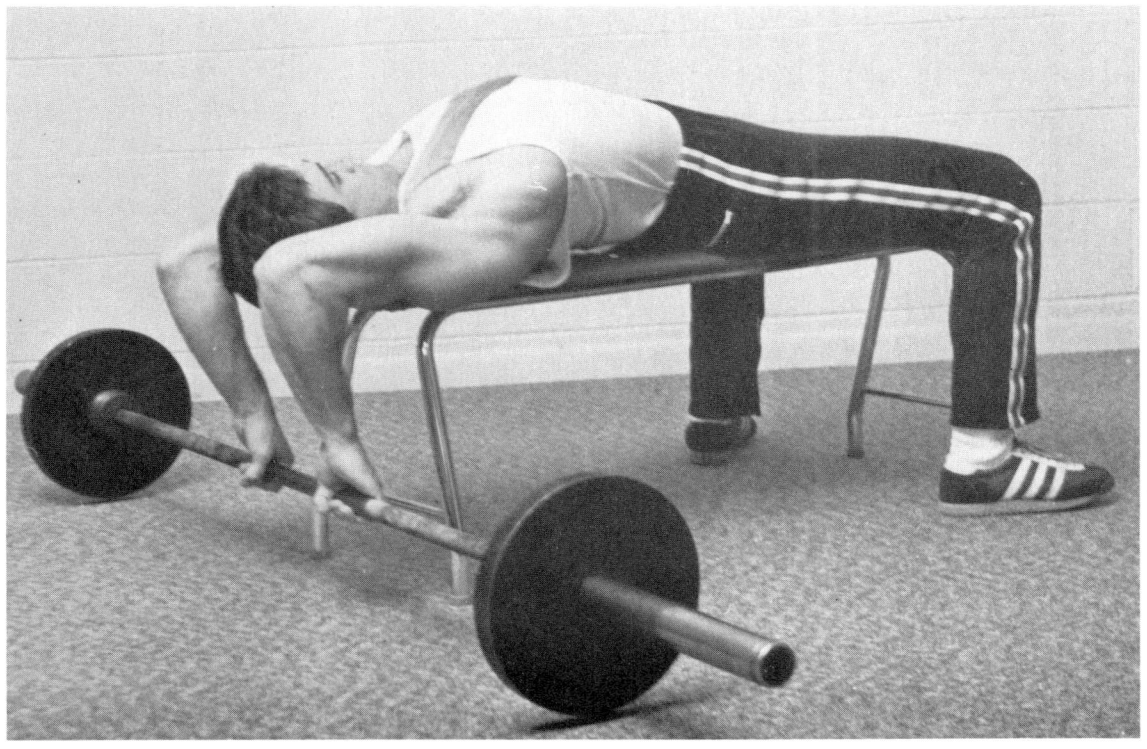

THE BENT-ARM PULLOVER begins as shown in the photo, the bar passing close to the head and face as it is pulled over to touch the upper chest and then returned to the starting position.

two dumbbells, you should hold them naturally at your sides, palms toward your legs at the start. As you flex your arms to bring the dumbbells to your shoulders, turn your hands toward a palms-up position so that your palms are toward your shoulders and the dumbbells are pointing end-to-end at the finish of the curling motion. Reverse the rotation as you lower the weights. Turning the palms up (supination) contributes to full contraction of the biceps.

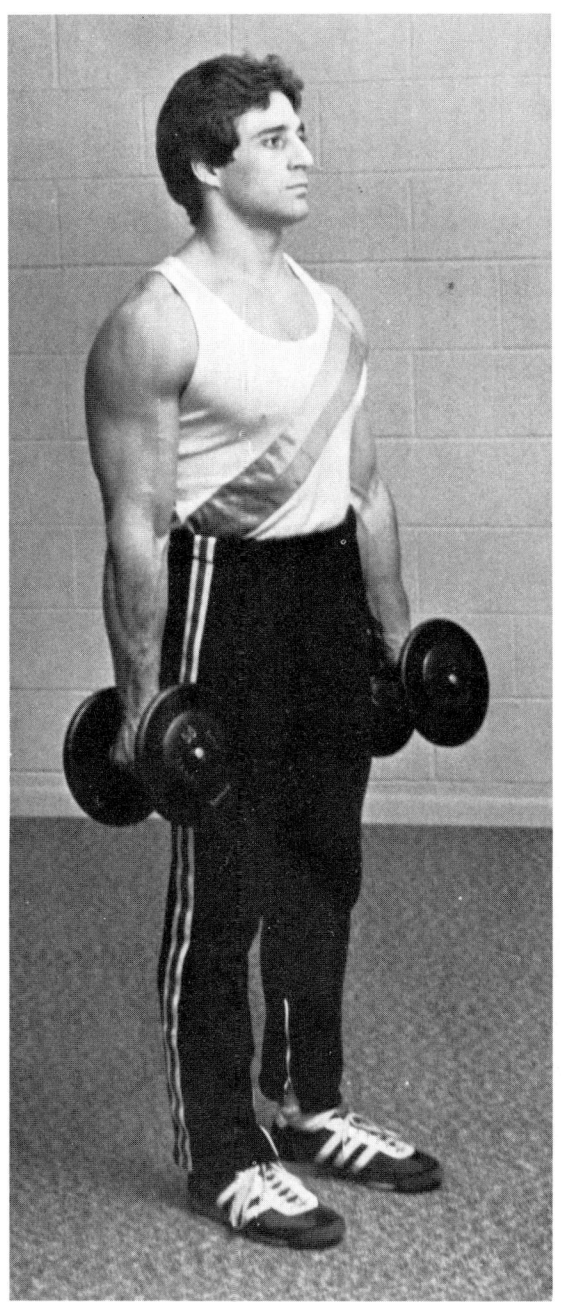 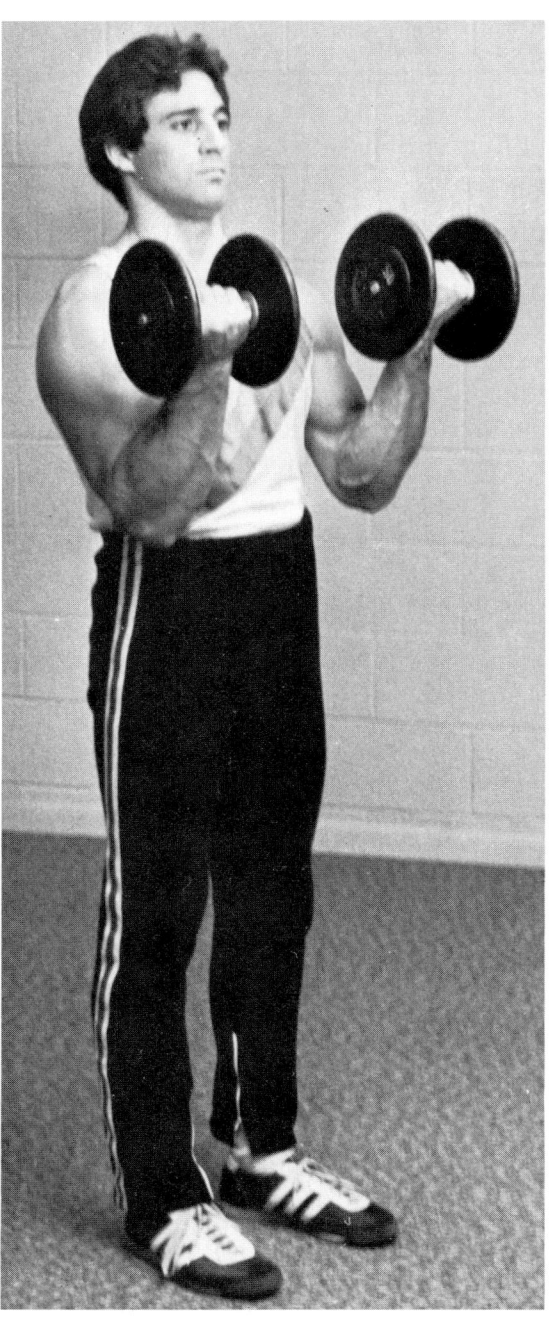

DUMBBELL CURLS are especially effective arm builders because they allow a natural rotation of the hands as the arms are flexed.

Dumbbell curls should be done eight to twelve reps, three sets. This exercise is not one to be added to the barbell curl, but rather it is a substitute for it—for the stimulation that comes from adding variety to your workouts. Dumbbell curls are especially convenient when you exercise at a gym where fixed-weight dumbbells of various poundages are readily available. It takes twice as long to change the weights of dumbbells as it does to change a barbell when training at home.

The "Concentration Curl"

A dumbbell curl that can be added to regular barbell curls or heavy two-dumbbell curls is the "concentration curl." This is done with a single dumbbell while either leaning forward or seated. Most exercisers prefer to sit on a bench, leaning forward and holding a dumbbell just off the floor. Brace the exercising arm against the inside of the thigh to minimize extraneous motion, such as swinging. The idea is to curl the dumbbell to your shoulder, all the while concentrating on fully contracting the biceps. The motion should be smooth and controlled, and you should do two or three sets of eight to twelve with each arm.

The Reverse Curl

A beginner to bodybuilding will obtain considerable exercise for his forearm muscles by holding onto the bar during such exercises as the curl and rowing

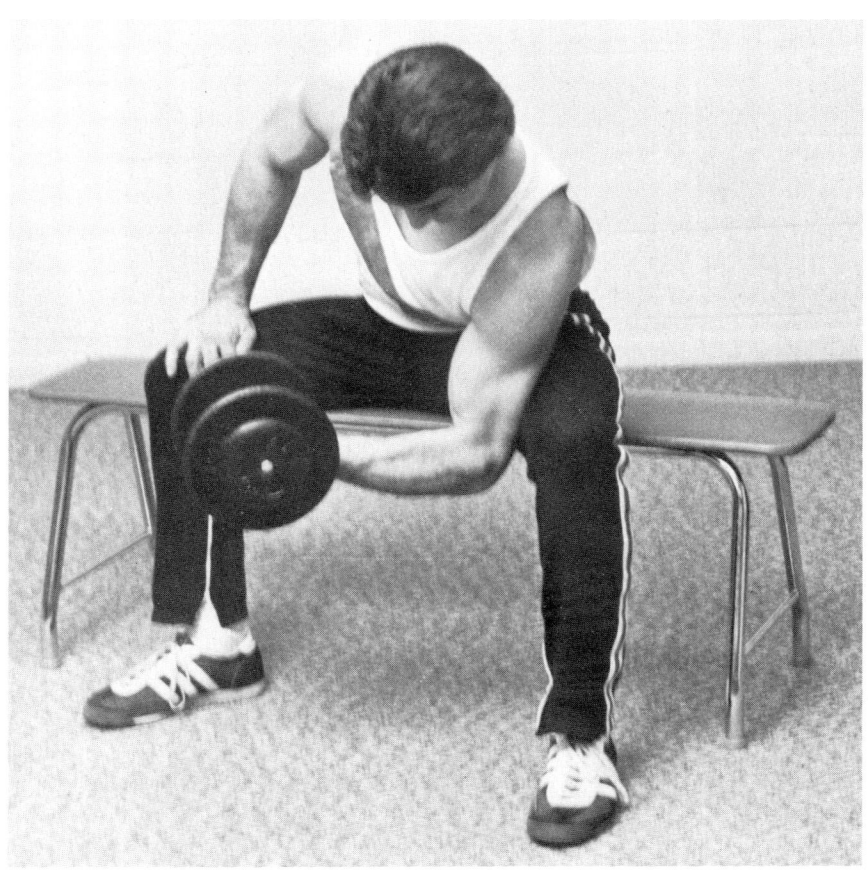

THE "CONCENTRATION CURL," as shown, is effective for developing a high peak on the biceps.

motion. But the forearm muscles can be exercised directly, and this will not only increase their size but also add strength to your grip and power to any movement that requires wrist action, such as swinging a baseball bat, tennis racquet, or golf club.

One good forearm exercise is the reverse curl, in which you perform a barbell curl, but with an overhand grip instead of a palms-up grip. For more intense forearm involvement, cock your hands toward your thighs at the start of the reverse curl, and then immediately cock your wrists up as you begin the upward curling motion.

You should do one to three sets of eight to twelve reps of the reverse curl, in which you will not be able to handle as much weight as in the regular curl. The heaviest weights lifted in single reverse curls are 20 percent or more lighter than the best regular curls done in good form.

The Wrist Curl

The forearm muscles can be isolated and worked intensively in an exercise known as the wrist curl. In this one, you sit holding a light barbell, with your forearms supported on your thighs; or you may kneel with your forearms supported across a bench. With your arms thus immobilized, raise and lower the barbell (or dumbbells) through as much range of motion as the mobility of your wrists will permit. This exercise should be done one to three sets of ten to fifteen reps with palms up and palms down.

A forearm exercise such as the reverse curl or wrist curl can be inserted into your training routine right after regular curls.

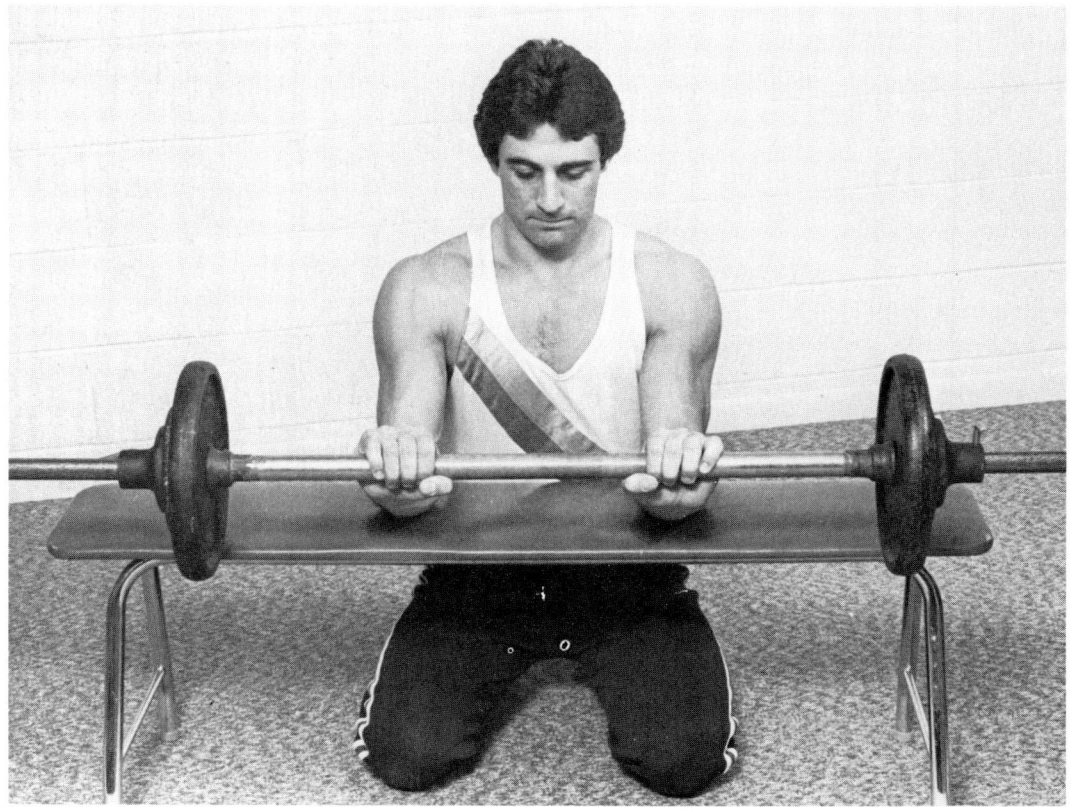

WRIST CURLS isolate the forearm muscles. The exercise should be done two ways—with knuckles up, as shown, and with palms up.

RISE-ON-TOES (SEATED)

The rise-on-toes exercise is the key exercise for the calf muscles, one of the basic movements, but it tends to focus action on the gastrocnemius, which is the large bulge of the calf near the knee. If you want to direct the exercise to the soleus muscle, which underlies the gastrocnemius and covers the lower part of the calf nearer the heel, you need to do the exercise with your knees bent. This calls for performing the exercise seated, with the barbell across your thighs near the knees. Obviously, you will have to place a thick pad under the bar to keep it from hurting your legs.

Do the seated version of this exercise with the balls of your feet elevated on a board, as when you do the rise-on-toes, standing. Concentrate on full stretch and contraction of the calf muscles. Less weight is required for this variation of the exercise, but use as much as you can handle comfortably and still go through the full range of motion.

"Donkey Calf Raise"

Another variation of the rise-on-toes calls for the cooperation of a training partner, preferably a heavy one. For this exercise, called the "donkey calf raise," stand with the balls of your feet elevated and lean forward from the hips, bracing your arms on a bench. Then have your training partner sit on your back while you perform the rise-on-toes motion from ten to twenty reps. You can do this exercise with your legs straight, to work the gastrocnemius, and with your knees bent slightly to involve the soleus more strongly.

ABDOMINAL EXERCISE

The Leg-Raise

There are many effective exercises for the mid-section in addition to the basic

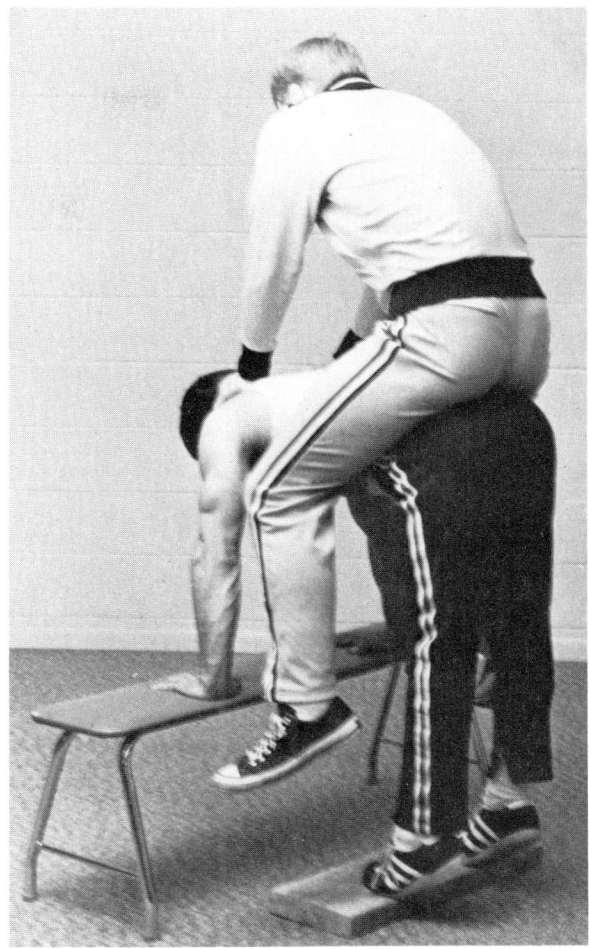

THE "DONKEY CALF RAISE" can be done with legs straight for the gastrocnemius (upper calf) and with knees bent for the soleus (lower calf).

crunch-type sit-up. One of the best is the leg-raise, in which you lie supine on a bench or the floor, hands gripping the bench or braced alongside your hips for balance, and raise your legs to point straight up. As with sit-ups, you may be able to focus the exercise on abdominal muscles and relax the thigh muscles and the deep-lying psoas (running from your thigh to your low back) by bending your knees slightly. To accentuate the effect on abdominal muscles, tense and draw them in deliberately as you raise your legs. Work up to ten to twenty repetitions or more (most advanced bodybuilders do at least fifty).

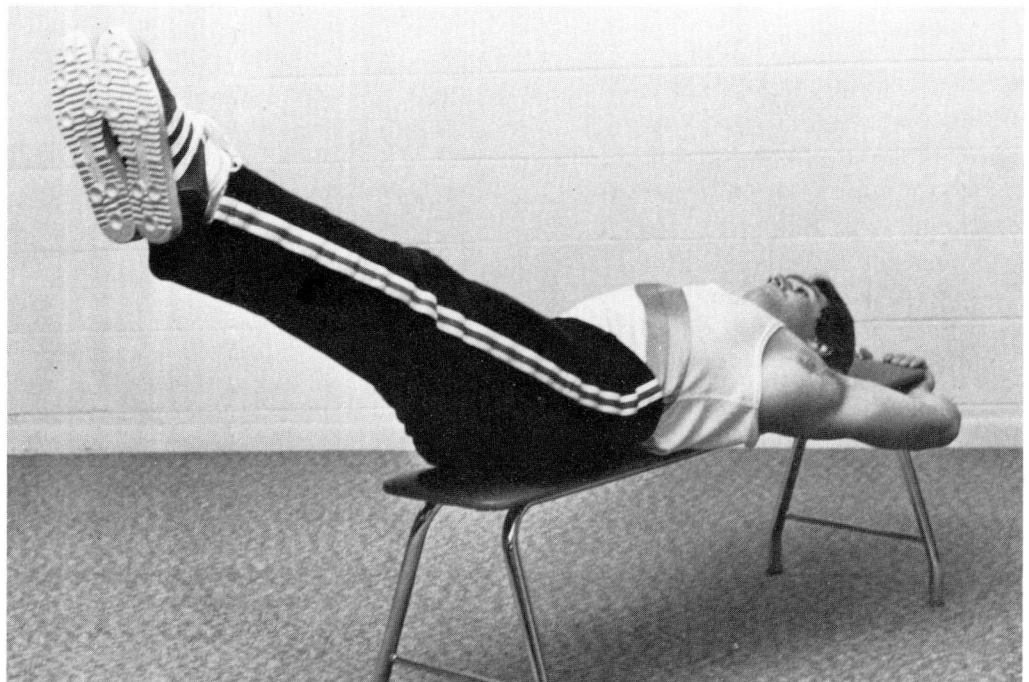

THE LEG-RAISE is an effective exercise for developing the abdominal muscles, especially the lower section. *(Below)* Twists work the sides of the waist vigorously. The feet should be anchored as shown to keep the hips from rotating with the upper body.

Twists

Another effective waistline exercise is the twist, done while holding an unloaded bar across your shoulders. With the bar across your shoulders and your arms stretched out along it, twist as far as you can first to one side then to the other, rotating your torso while keeping your hips as stationary as possible. One way to keep your hips stationary is to sit on a bench. Another effective way to do twists is to lean forward from your hips and twist your torso first to one side and then to the other as though you were alternately touching your toes. Twisting exercises should be done in high repetitions, working up to twenty-five to each side for a total of fifty. Advanced bodybuilders do many more.

Knee-Ups

A particularly effective exercise for the abdominal muscles requires either a steeply slanted abdominal board or something that will serve as a chinning bar. If

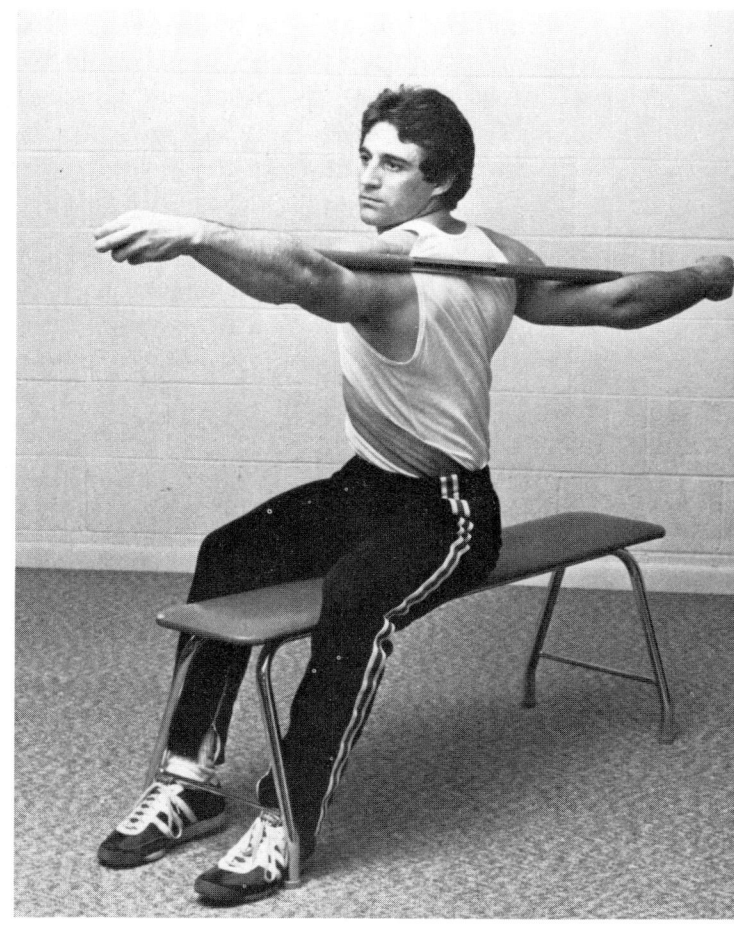

you have a chinning bar that is located high enough so that you can hang from it without your feet touching the floor, perform a knee-up from the hang, attempting to touch your knees to your chest. Bend your knees as you pull them up, and then straighten your legs as you lower them. The same exercise can be done on a slant board, and it is a bit easier that way because your back is supported and the leverage is changed somewhat. Either way, however, this is a difficult exercise, so a good goal is to work gradually to ten to twenty repetitions.

the sides of the waistline. For this one, you need the help of a training partner or access to a special exercise bench known as a "Roman chair for sit-ups and hyperextensions." In either case, you assume a prone position with your legs supported to the upper thighs; the training partner, or the padded piece of a Roman chair, presses down on your ankles. In this position, with your upper body extending out from the bench, clasp your hands behind your neck, lower your torso until your head almost touches the floor, and then arch up as high as you can. In the arched

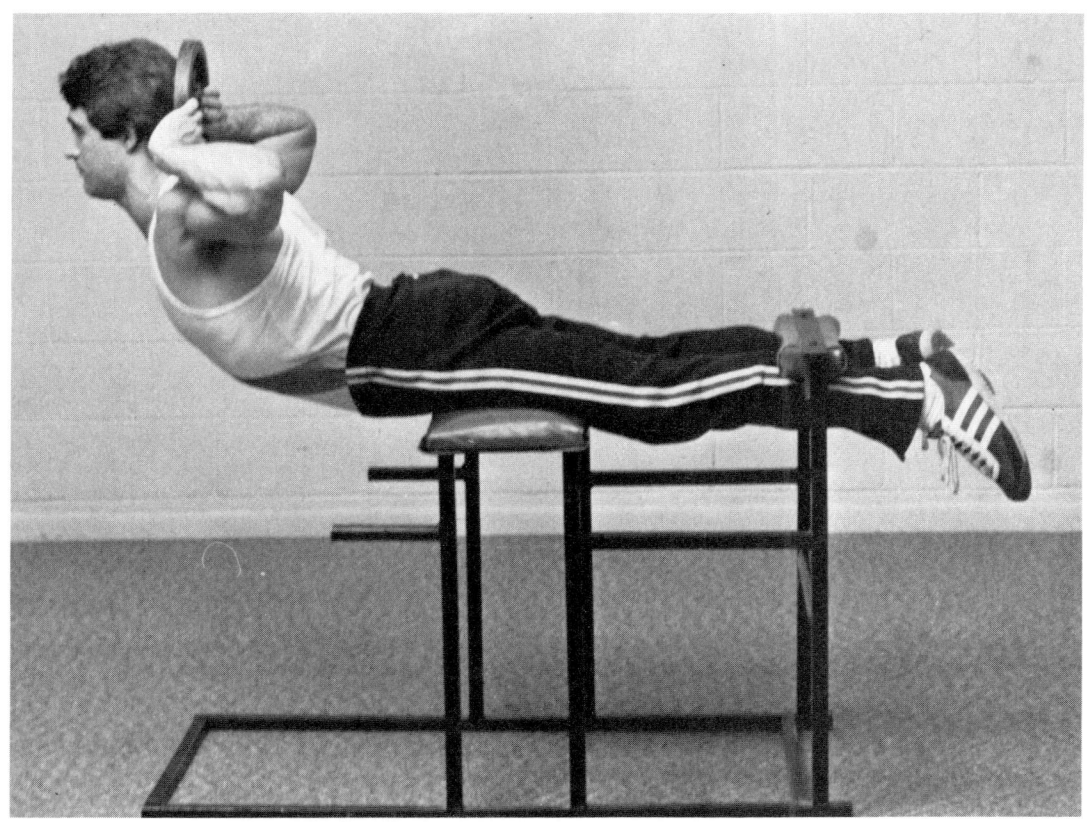

THE HYPEREXTENSION is the most effective exercise for working the low back muscles, especially when weight is held behind the neck, as shown.

HYPEREXTENSION

A hyperextension movement, done like a reverse sit-up in the prone position, is one of the best exercises for the low back area, and it also can be used to exercise

(hyperextended) position, your head and shoulders should be higher than your buttocks.

Do five to ten hyperextensions to start, and then work up gradually until you can do ten to twenty. When it becomes easy to do ten to twenty, hold a 5-pound weight behind your head. A good goal is to be able to do ten to fifteen hyperextensions with 25 pounds or more behind your head. This exercise develops the low back muscles that run alongside the spine.

To work the muscles of your sides and back simultaneously, arch up into a hyperextended position and then swing your head and shoulders alternately as far to the left and right as you can. This exercise should be done ten to twenty repetitions or more. Added weight is not needed for the side-to-side version.

In the eight exercises of the basic workout, the low back muscles receive benefit from holding an erect position in the squat and also are strengthened in the performance of the bent-over rowing motion. Hyperextensions can be added to the basic routine after either the rowing exercise or the sit-up.

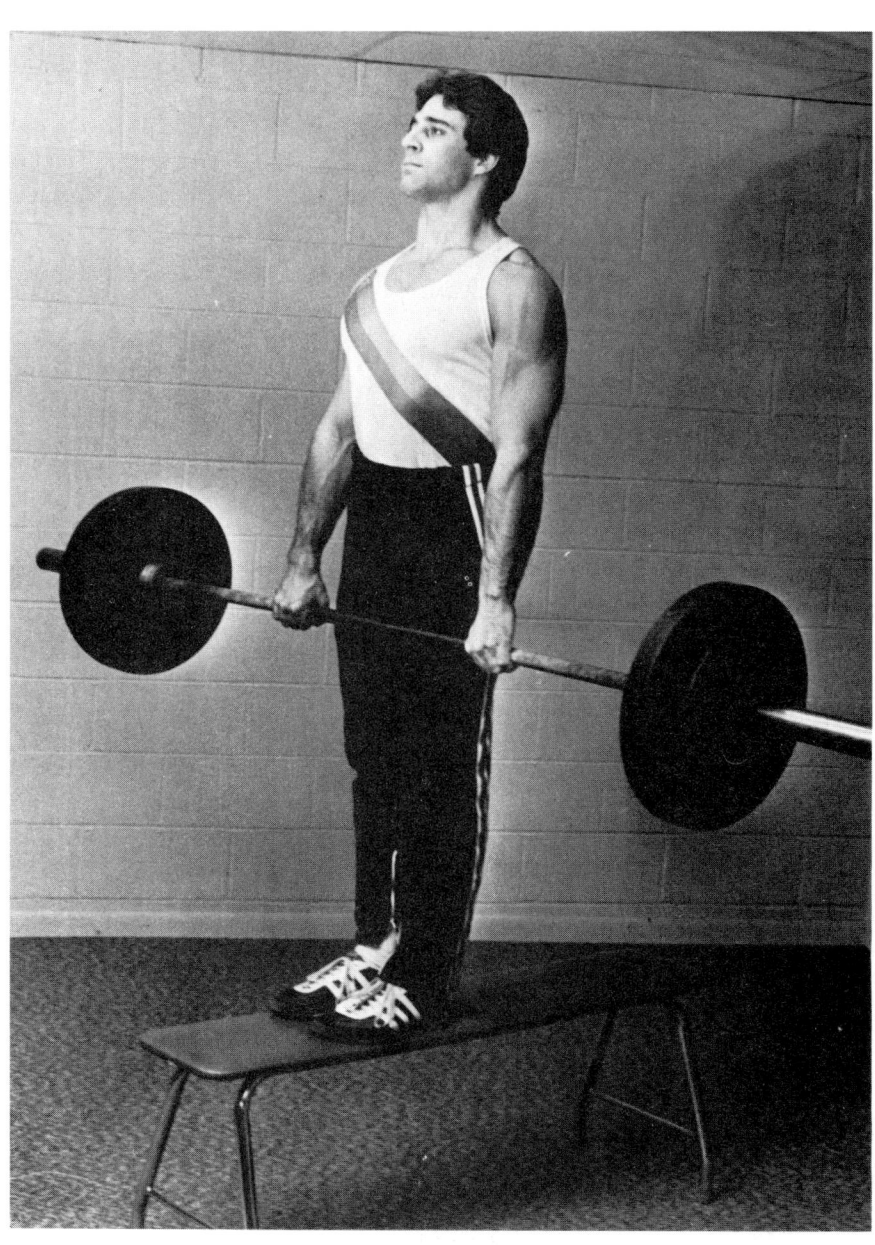

THE STIFF-LEGGED DEAD LIFT (shown here and on the next page) strengthens the back and keeps it flexible, but it should be done only with caution—as described in the text.

STIFF-LEGGED DEAD LIFT

Another good low back exercise, providing you do not have a "touchy" low back that is prone to strain, is the stiff-legged dead lift. In this exercise, pick up the barbell either with an overhand grip or with one hand in the overhand position and the other reversed, palm away (reversing the hands aids your grip, countering any tendency for the barbell to "roll" out of your fingers.) Stand with the barbell hanging across your thighs. Then, keeping your legs straight or very slightly bent, bend forward, touch the weight to the floor, and straighten again. In other words, the exercise is like toe-touching with a barbell in your hands.

If you work into the stiff-legged dead lift carefully, starting with light weights in order to get used to the stretch without strain, the exercise is one of the best for thickening the muscles that run along the spine on either side. When your back becomes strong and flexible, you can add to the effectiveness of the exercise by standing on a box or bench and stretching to touch your knuckles to the tops of your feet as you hold the bar.

Thirty pounds is plenty of weight to start with in the stiff-legged dead lift, but someone who is strong and fit might start with more, perhaps 50 to 100 pounds. It isn't necessary to use heavy weights in this exercise. A strong man can get a good workout for his low back muscles with 150 pounds, but advanced bodybuilders have used 400 pounds and more. Some

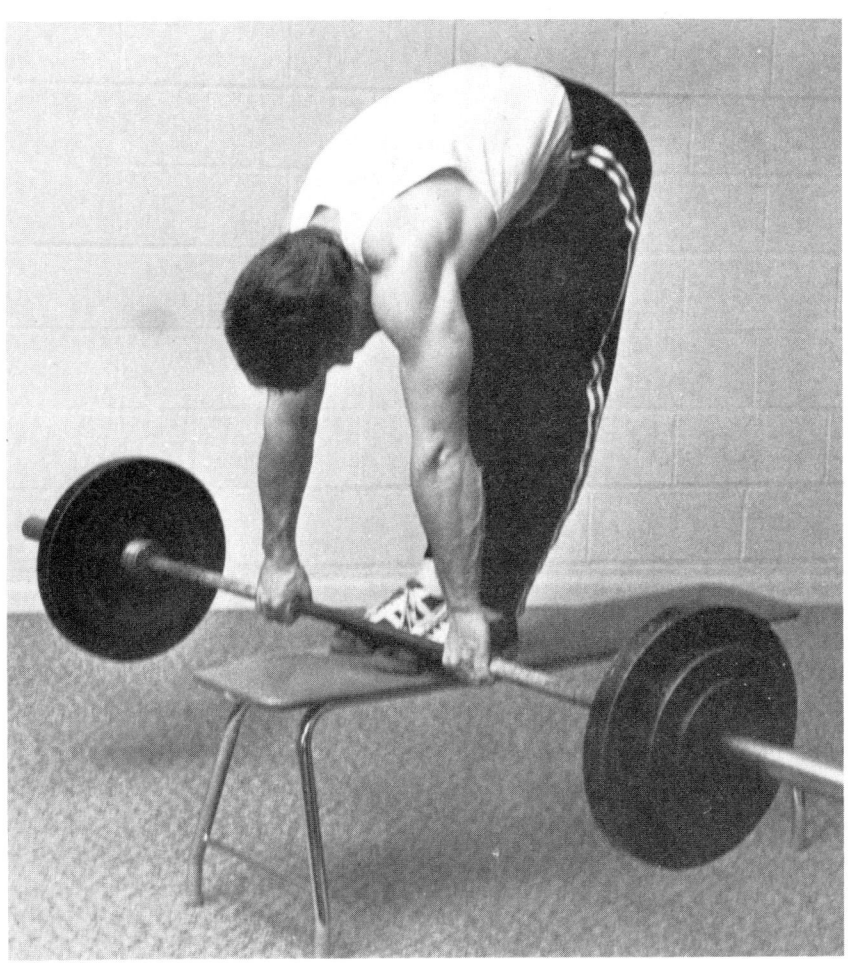

people have structural inadequacy of the low back that makes them prone to painful strains from lifting with a rounded back. If you suspect that you have this problem, do not do stiff-legged dead lifts, and always be particularly careful to keep a flat back when rowing, squatting, cleaning a weight to your chest, and even when picking up a weight to do an exercise such as the curl.

VARIETIES OF TRICEPS EXTENSIONS

I mentioned previously that the triceps muscles at the backs of the arms contribute much more muscular bulk than the biceps. It is more difficult to get the feel of working the triceps than the biceps, however, which is probably why various curls are more popular than triceps exercises. To work the triceps thoroughly, you must isolate the muscle, and this can be done in several ways.

"French Press"

One of the best triceps extensions is the so-called "French press." This is an over-

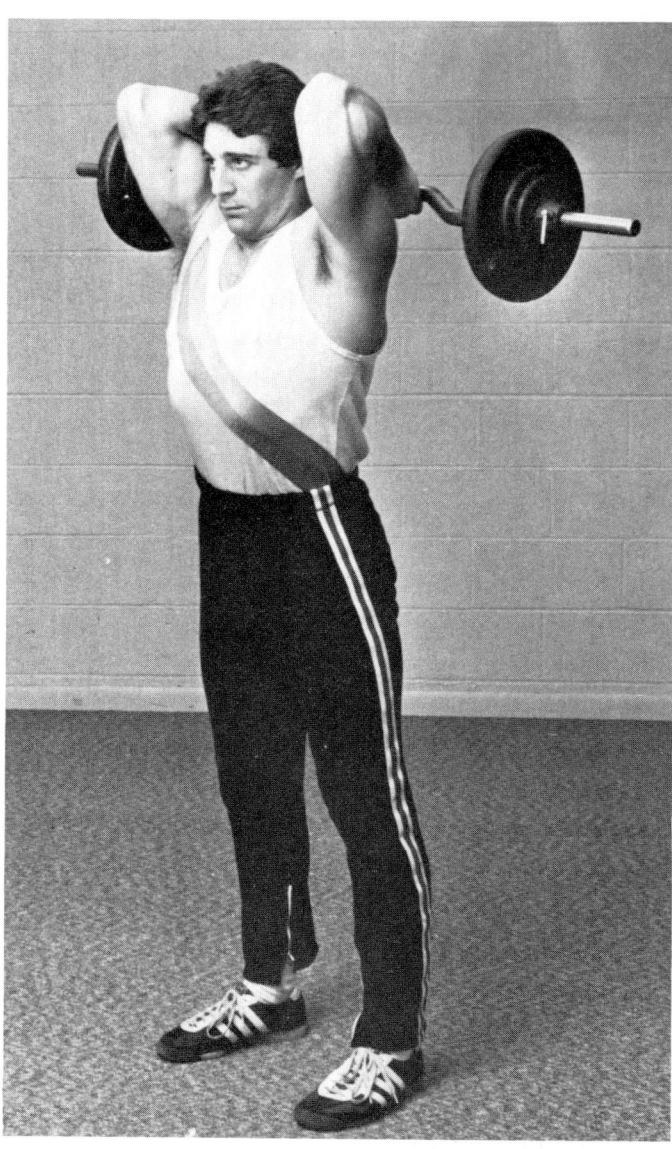

THE TRICEPS EXTENSION, STANDING, or "French press" (shown here and on the next page) is one of the best ways to exercise the triceps from a fully stretched position. The elbows should point straight up throughout.

head triceps extension, done with a narrow, overhand grip on a barbell or with two hands on a single dumbbell. It also can be done one arm at a time with a lighter dumbbell.

With a barbell, your grip should place your hands close enough to each other so that your thumbs, if extended along the bar, would touch. Hold the barbell over-head and—keeping your elbows pointed straight up—lower it in an arc to the back of your neck. Immediately force it back up until your arms are straight, still keeping your upper arms pointing up alongside your head. Work in the range of eight to twelve reps, up to three sets.

A variation of this is to do the exercise while lying supine on a bench. Again,

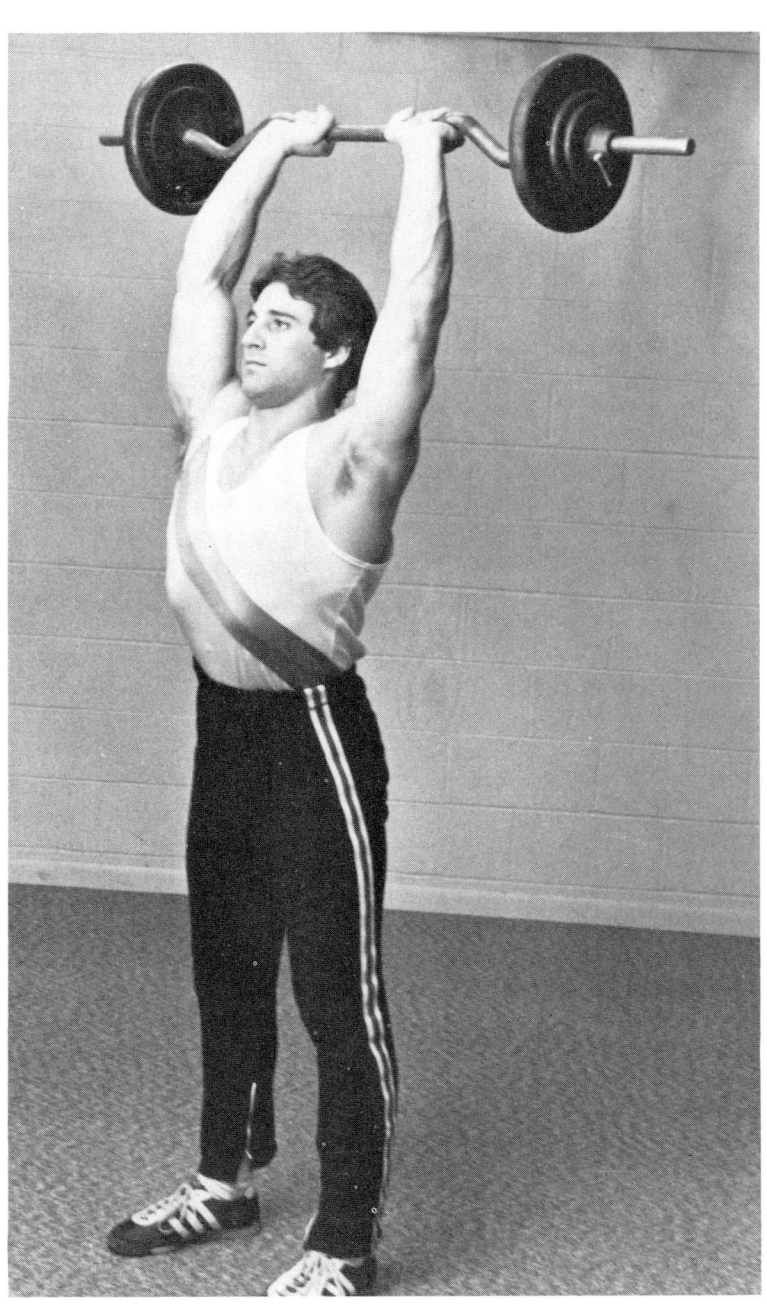

your elbows point up throughout. Lower the weight to touch your forehead (lightly!), and force it back up to straight arms. This exercise can be done with two dumbbells, which are lowered alongside your head to touch your shoulders before being forced back to straight arms. Work in the eight to twelve range for three sets.

Triceps Kick-back

When you do the triceps extension lying supine, you can maintain continuous tension on the muscles by tilting your upper arms slightly toward your head and keeping them in that position rather than pointing straight up. But an even more effective, continuous-tension exercise is

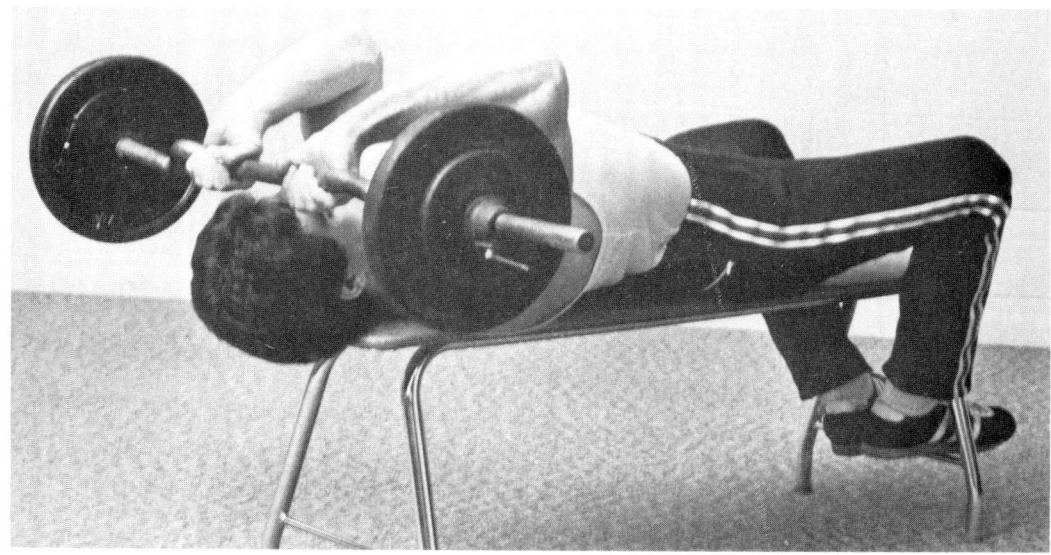

IN THE SUPINE POSITION, continuous tension can be maintained on the triceps by pointing the elbows up but tilted slightly toward the head throughout the extension movement.

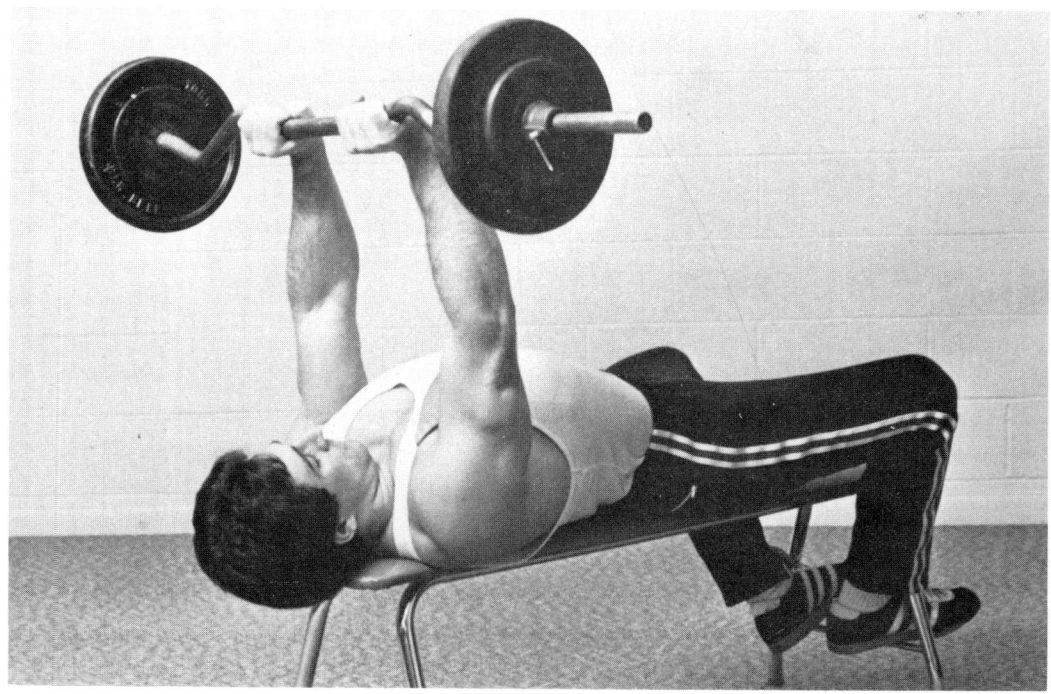

the triceps kick-back, done with two dumbbells or, more often, with a single dumbbell, one arm at a time. (Kick-backs also can be done effectively with a pulley, if you have access to a floor-level pulley device at a gymnasium.)

To do the triceps kick-back, hold a dumbbell (or two dumbbells) and bend forward from the hips until your back is horizontal (knees slightly bent for comfort). Bend your arm (arms) as though you had just completed a curl, keeping your upper arm(s) along your body (also horizontal). Then, trying to move nothing but your arm(s) from the elbow(s) to the

dumbbell(s) you are holding, straighten your arm(s) fully.

When your arm(s) is straight (horizontal, the same as your body), try to raise the dumbbell(s) higher, allowing your upper arm(s) to move for the first time. At this point, you should feel a distinct cramp in your triceps, and the effectiveness of the exercise will be evident. After briefly raising the dumbbell(s) to this highest point, bring it (them) back to the starting point, moving your upper arm(s) down only enough to bring it (them) back in line with your body.

If you do the triceps kick-back right,

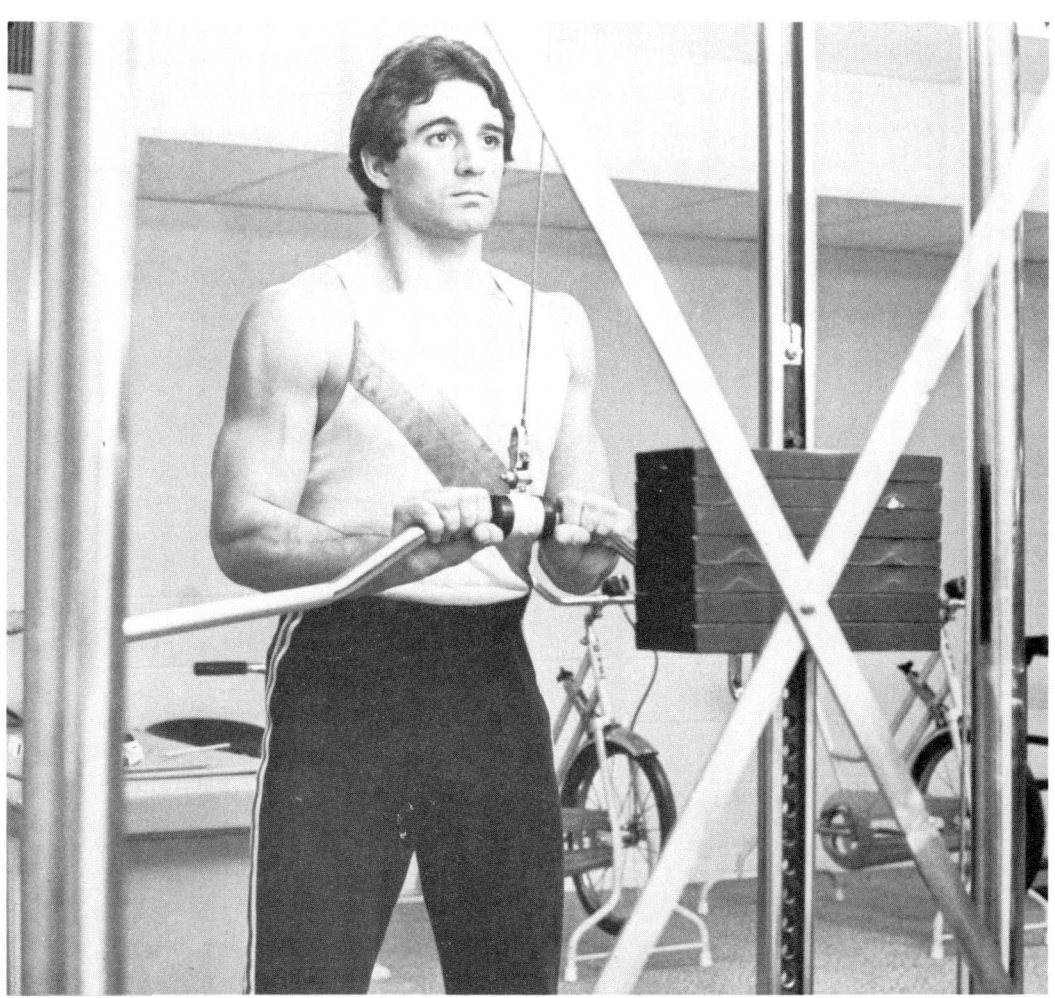

THE PUSH-DOWN, an excellent triceps builder, can be performed on a lat machine. A close grip is best, and the elbows should be kept immobile at the sides, as shown.

you won't need much weight. Experiment with a 15-pound dumbbell and adjust the weight so ten to twelve reps feel like enough, but not too much work.

Triceps Push-down

Another excellent triceps builder is the triceps push-down, which requires access to a lat machine. In this exercise you grasp the lat machine bar in an overhand grip with narrow hand spacing and, keeping your elbows at your sides, straighten your arms so the bar travels in an arc from your chest to your thighs. Three sets of eight to twelve reps should produce good results.

The triceps exercises (one or two of them) should be added to your workout after curls.

PRESS BEHIND NECK

All overhead presses develop the shoulders, primarily the front part (anterior deltoid) and to some extent the side

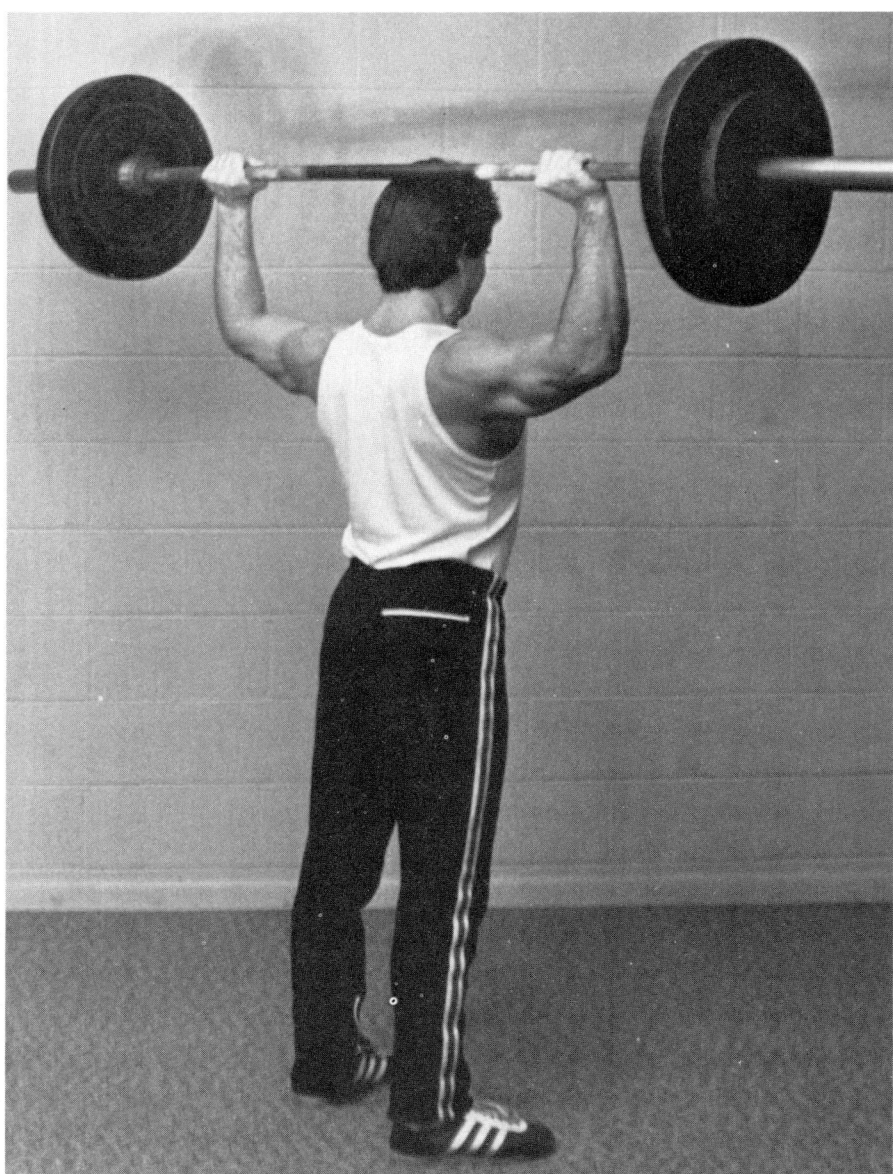

THE PRESS BEHIND NECK is a favorite shoulder-developer for many bodybuilders.

(lateral deltoid), and the triceps of the back of the upper arm. A variation of the barbell press is to take a slightly wider grip than you would use for the regular press and lower the barbell to touch low at the back of your neck. This is called the press behind neck and is an especially good shoulder developer. Three sets of eight to twelve reps should be effective. You will not be able to use as much weight when pressing behind the neck as when doing the regular front press.

Dumbbell Press

Another press variation that is a good shoulder developer is to do the above exercise with two dumbbells. Dumbbells are always effective pieces of equipment because they force each arm to do as much work as the other. To do the exercise, clean the dumbbells to your shoulders, and then turn them so that the dumbbell bars point straight out to the sides. Your elbows should be out to the

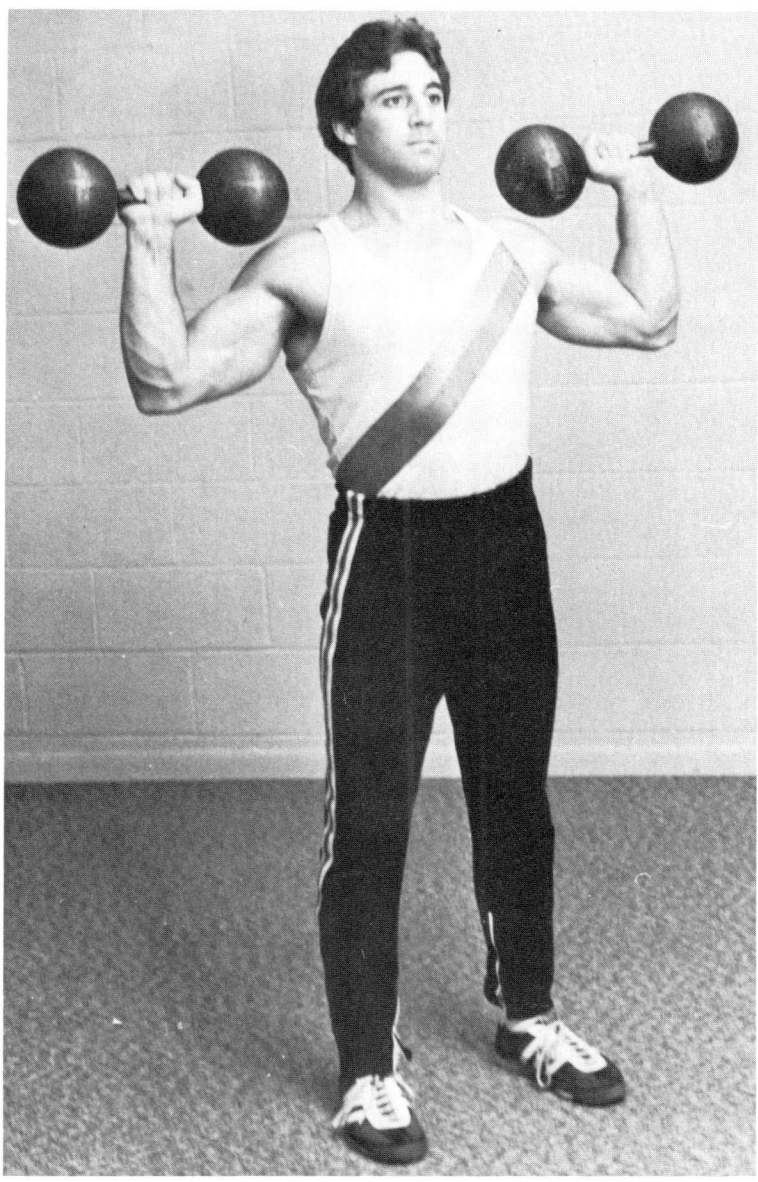

DUMBBELL PRESSES should be done with arms well out to the sides and dumbbell handles pointing straight outward. This permits a strong activation of the deltoid muscles.

sides, and the insides of the dumbbells should just touch the outer edges of your shoulders.

Push the dumbbells straight up and lower them to the starting position for eight to twelve repetitions, three sets. Many exercisers like to do the dumbbell press alternately, one dumbbell coming down as the other goes up, but this encourages excessive body motion that takes work away from the shoulder and arm muscles you are trying to develop.

Unless you are a very serious bodybuilder who thrives on hard work, the press behind neck and dumbbell press are substitutes for, not additions to, the regular barbell press in your workout.

DUMBBELL RAISES

Although overhead pressing exercises are excellent shoulder developers, the exercises that work the deltoid muscles most directly are leverage movements with relatively light dumbbells. The anterior, or

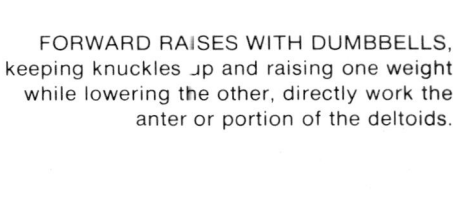

FORWARD RAISES WITH DUMBBELLS, keeping knuckles up and raising one weight while lowering the other, directly work the anter or portion of the deltoids.

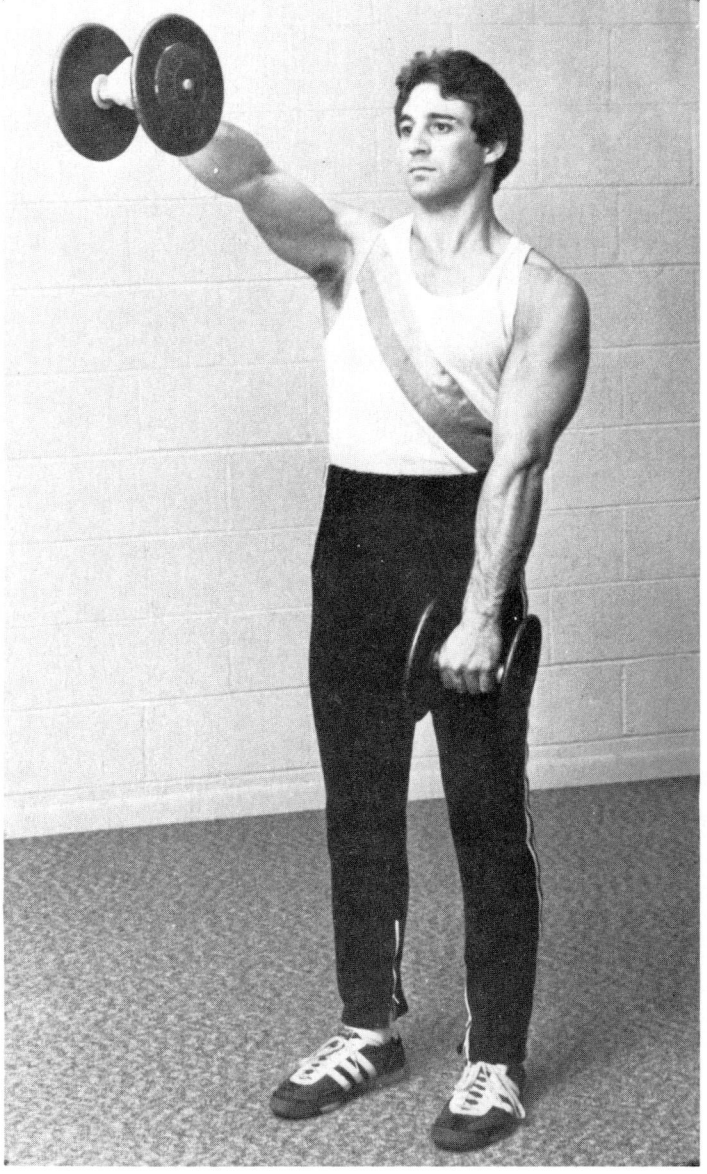

front, section of the deltoid raises the arm forward, the lateral section raises the arm to the side, and the posterior, or back, section raises the arm backward (pulls it up and back) when you are leaning forward.

To work the fronts of the deltoids, hold a pair of dumbbells at the fronts of your thighs, arms hanging almost straight (but with elbows unlocked), and raise and lower the arms alternately in an arc in front of your body, starting at the thigh and ending with the dumbbell fully overhead. As soon as one dumbbell is overhead, begin to lower it while simultaneously raising the other one. Continue for twenty repetitions, ten with each arm. If you do the exercise strictly, you can derive benefit from working with 10- or 15-pound dumbbells, but it is possible to handle considerably more as your shoulders get stronger. It also is possible to handle more weight by increasing the bend in your arms and swinging the

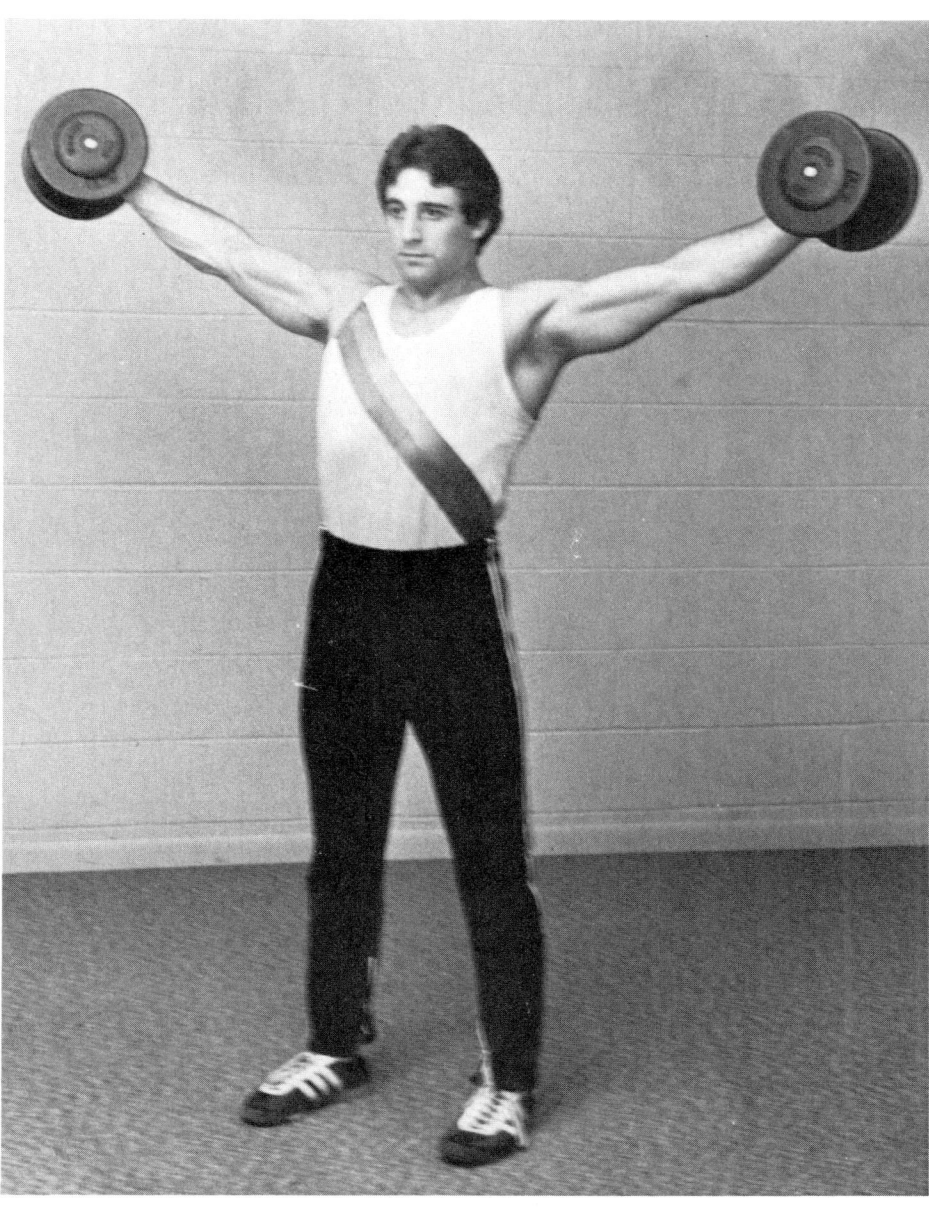

TO FOCUS the work of raising dumbbells on the side (lateral) portions of the deltoids, the front ends of the dumbbells should tilt slightly downward (more than is shown in the picture).

weights up with the help of body motion. Most advanced bodybuilders cheat in this way, and it's all right to do so as long as you are able to feel the deltoid working.

To work the sides of the deltoids, hold a pair of dumbbells at your sides, arms hanging straight but elbows unlocked. Raise the weights simultaneously directly to each side, keeping your knuckles up as you elevate the weights to a point where they are at least as high as the top of your head. It is very important *not* to let your hands turn so that your thumbs point up as you raise the dumbbells. Your thumbs should be *down* throughout the movement. In fact, you should make an effort to keep the front ends of the dumbbells tilted slightly downward, which will focus the work on the lateral deltoids and not permit the anterior deltoids to take over. Do three sets of ten to twelve reps in the lateral raise.

To work the backs of the deltoids, lean well forward from the hips or lean in a prone position (face down) against an incline bench and perform lateral raises in

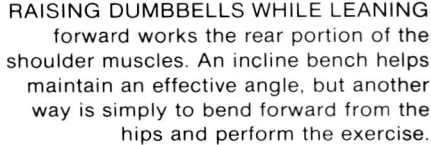

RAISING DUMBBELLS WHILE LEANING forward works the rear portion of the shoulder muscles. An incline bench helps maintain an effective angle, but another way is simply to bend forward from the hips and perform the exercise.

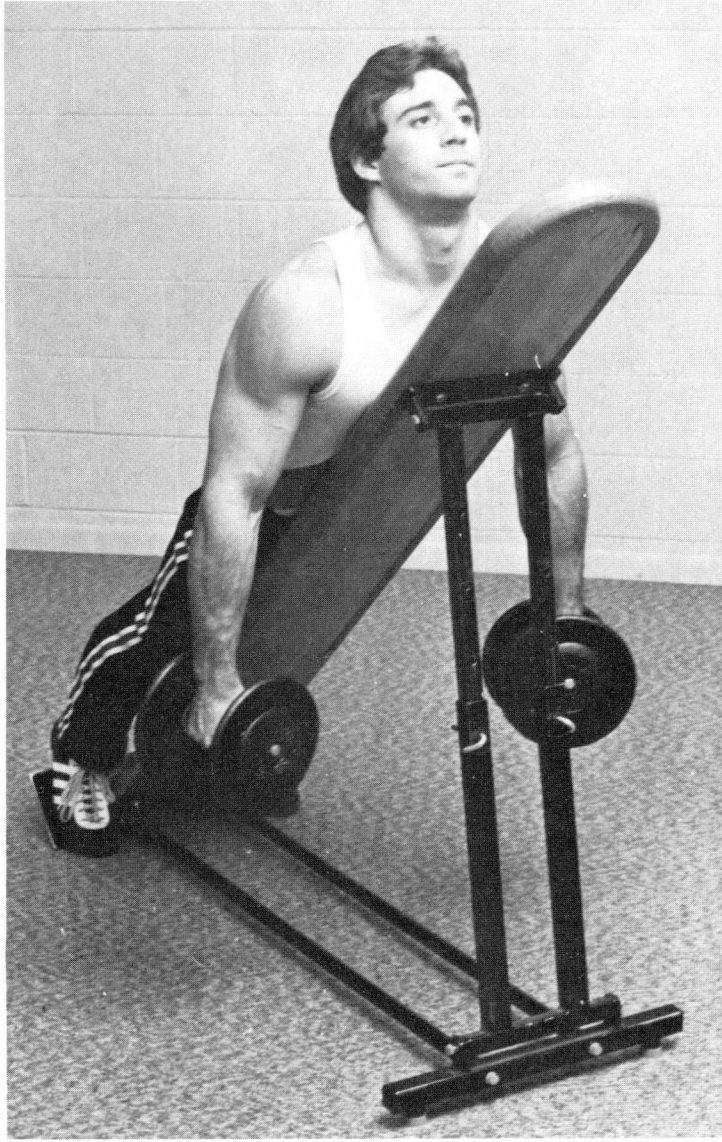

this position. The angle is important because the motion must be up and back, to the extent that the mobility of the shoulder joints permits. Try for a brief hold—a half-second at the highest point—to contract fully the portions of the posterior deltoids that this exercise works. You may find that you need a more pronounced bend of your arms to get the feel of this exercise than when you are doing the regular standing lateral raise, especially if you do the exercise face down against an incline bench. Do the lateral raise, leaning, three sets of ten to twelve reps.

SPECIAL EQUIPMENT

As much as possible, I've described body-building exercises that you can do with only the most basic equipment. You absolutely need a barbell, dumbbells, squat stands to hold the barbell at shoulder height, and a bench for supine presses and other exercises done lying down. It's possible to construct an incline bench with a sturdy board, braced so it won't slip.

Complete and advanced bodybuilding, however, calls for several pieces of special equipment that you can purchase for your home gym. You may find it more convenient to join a gym or health club where the equipment is available. It's also fun to work out at a club where you find others with similar interests.

Joining a Gym

Some of the very expensive "spa"-type

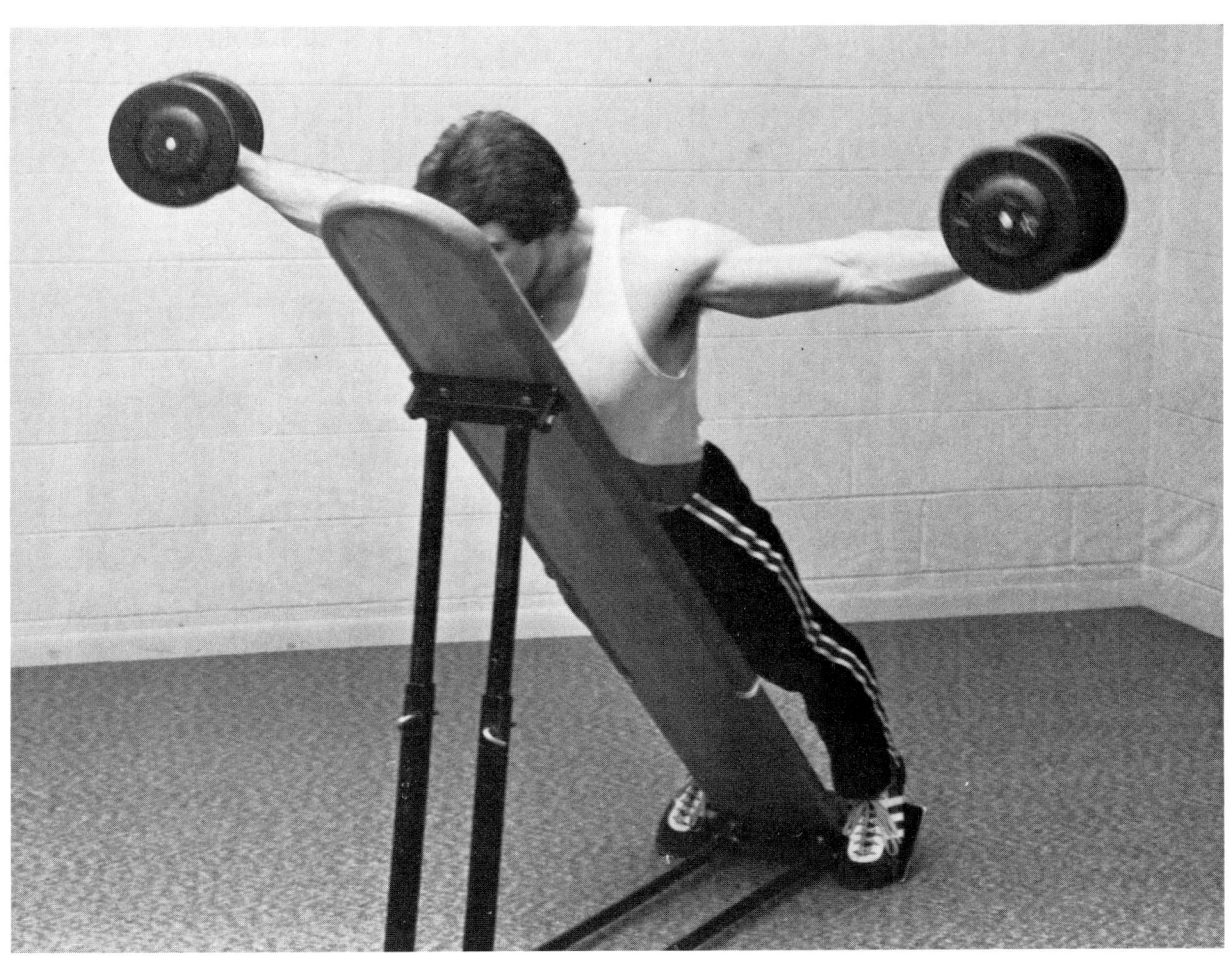

health clubs are more concerned with getting you to sign long-term contracts than with your welfare. You will be wise to investigate carefully and not join on the first visit unless you are absolutely certain that the membership costs are reasonable, and that the facilities and the essential pieces of equipment will be available when you want to use them.

At our club, the Bucks Fitness Center (for Bucks County, PA), there is no contract. We have a membership agreement that suggests you get a physical exam before exercising and points out that we take no responsibility for injuries: You only pay for the time and facilities you are going to use. Most clubs have reduced rates for longer-term memberships, as we do, so if you are serious about bodybuilding, you can probably save money by joining for an extended time. But be care-

ful about contracts. When you sign one, you are entering a binding legal agreement.

If you intend to join a gym, ask some of the present members how they like it and whether they would recommend that you join. In fact, that's a good way to locate a gym. If you learn that a compatible person is active in weight training, ask him (or her) where he (or she) works out. If such a person is satisfied with the gym, you probably will be, too. Working out at a good gym can be a relaxing social experience as well as physically beneficial.

Types of Equipment

Equipment that is especially useful and convenient includes fixed-weight dumbbells at various poundages so you don't waste time changing weights; slant boards for abdominal exercises (sit-ups, knee-

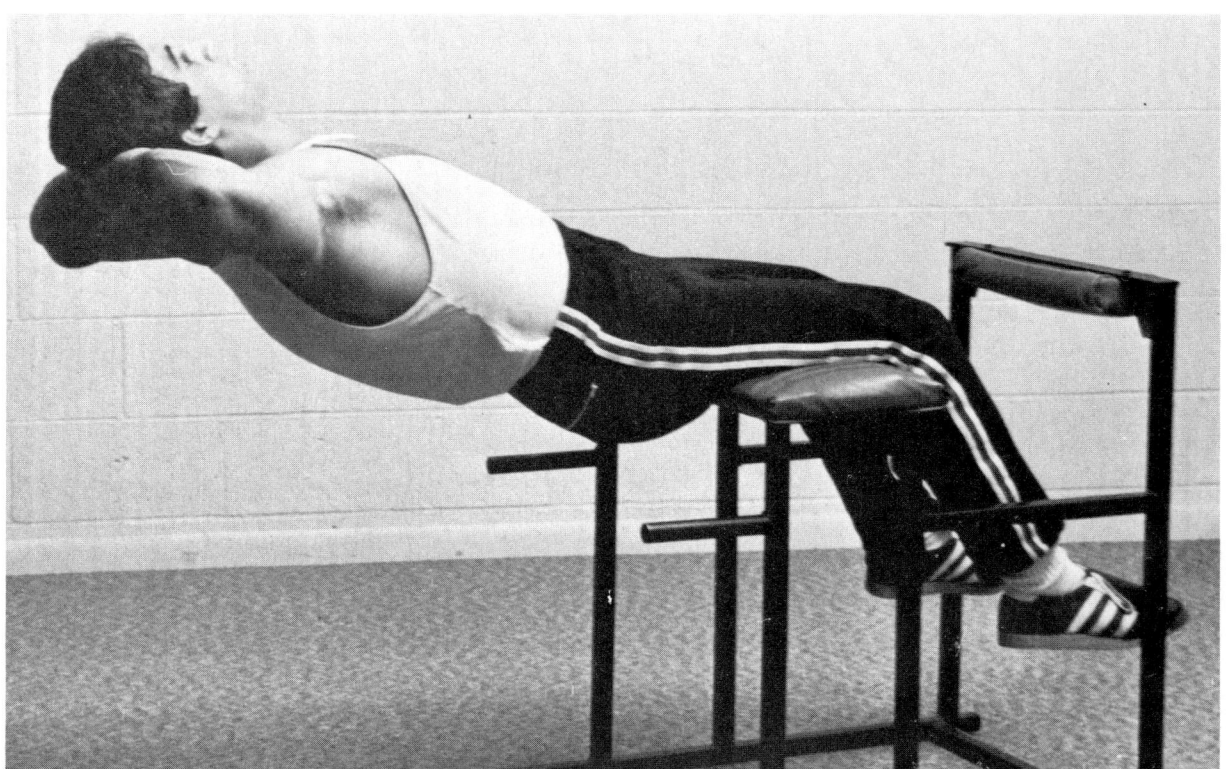

THE SAME "ROMAN CHAIR" that is used for hyperextensions can be used for a particularly effective sit-up variation. In this exercise the bodybuilder goes only as far back as shown and stops just short of sitting up straight to keep tension on the abdominal muscles.

ups, and leg-raises); overhead pulleys (lat machines) for latissimus pull-downs and triceps push-downs; low cable pulleys (for a particularly effective variation of rowing); incline benches for barbell and dumbbell presses, an effective variation of the dumbbell curl, the flying exercise, and the posterior deltoid raise; a "preacher bench" for high-intensity biceps work (curls); a Roman chair for sit-ups and hyperextensions; and machines for leg pressing (in which very heavy weights can be used to develop the thighs), leg curling (for thigh biceps), and leg extensions (a leverage movement for the thigh extensors).

A gym will probably also have additional cable apparatus for continuous-tension exercises, affecting muscles at their peak contraction point. Another **advantage** of a well-equipped gym is that there is usually some provision for purely aerobic exercise, so that you can top-off a workout with some work on a stationary bicycle or treadmill for cardiovascular effect. If you have an opportunity to do some outdoor jogging, you won't need this, but sometimes the weather will confine you to strictly indoor workouts.

Exercise Machines

Some gyms have very expensive exercise machines with cam and cable or chain rigs that apply continuous or peak contraction resistance to isolated muscles or muscle groups. Theoretically, these would seem to be very effective muscle-peakers for bodybuilding. I have tested one, made by Nautilus, that did produce a strong cramping sensation in the muscles being exercised.

Many leading bodybuilders say they

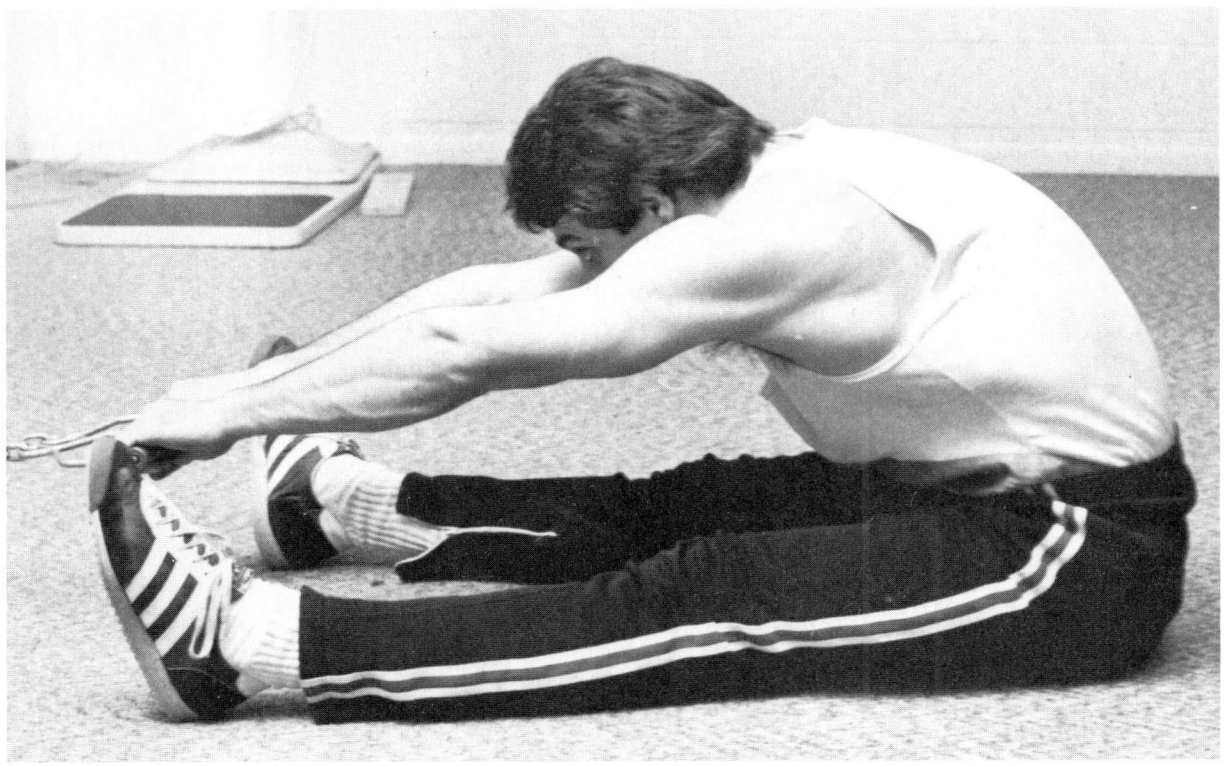

THE LOW CABLE ROW (shown here and on the next page) is one of the best exercises for the lower portion of the latissimus dorsi muscles. By leaning forward and pulling back, the muscles are worked from a fully stretched position.

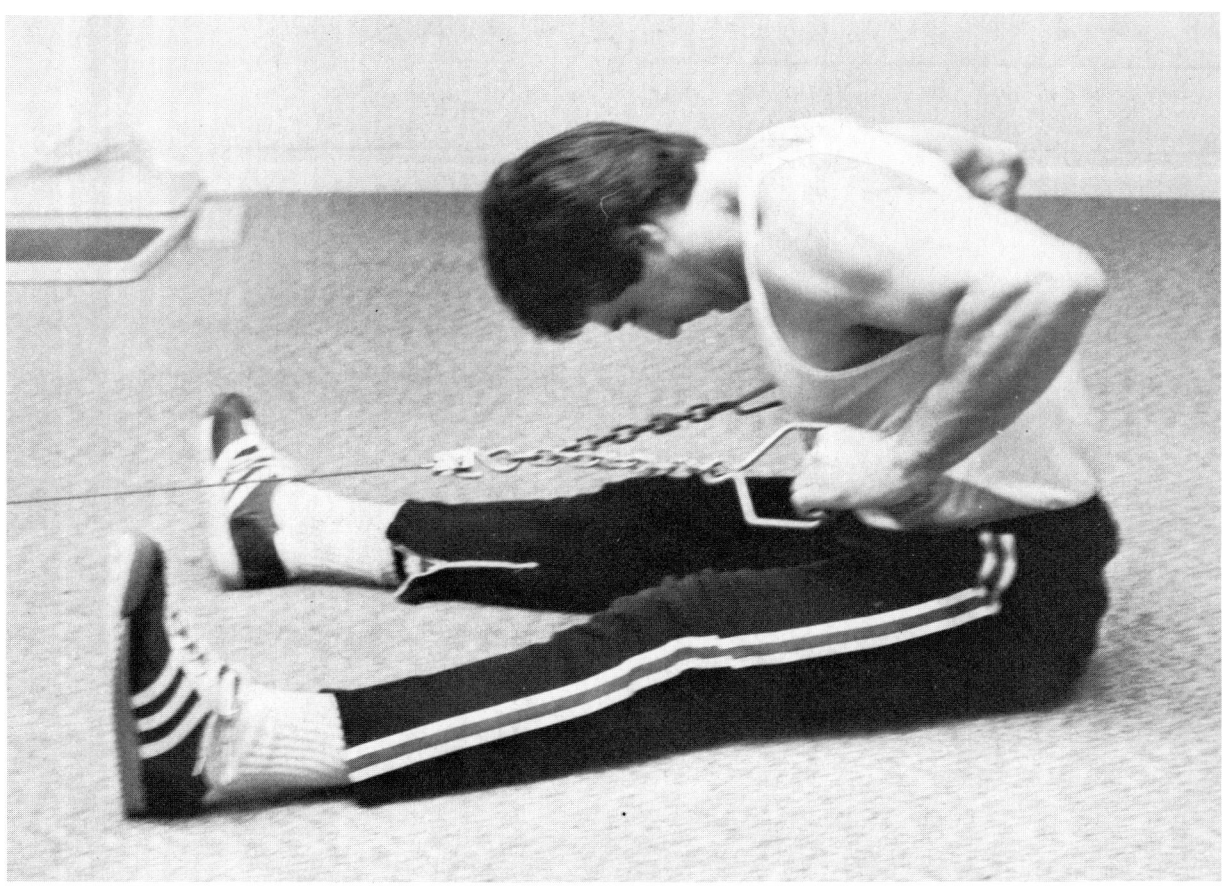

prefer to use standard equipment, however, and it may be that the intensity of exercise that these machines produce makes it impossible for a bodybuilder to continue exercising long enough to get the "pump" sensation that he seeks, in which the muscles are fully suffused with blood as well as fatigued from the work performed.

It seems to me that most pieces of special equipment have their place in a bodybuilding program, if you can gain access to them, but none of them actually can replace the basic items—barbell, dumbbells, benches, and squat stands—that have been fundamental in building all of the championship physiques of the past three decades and longer. Most men would be happy to match the muscular proportions developed by such bodybuilders as the famous Eugen Sandow, at the turn of the century, John Grimek, or Siegmund Klein, all of whom worked with only the most basic equipment.

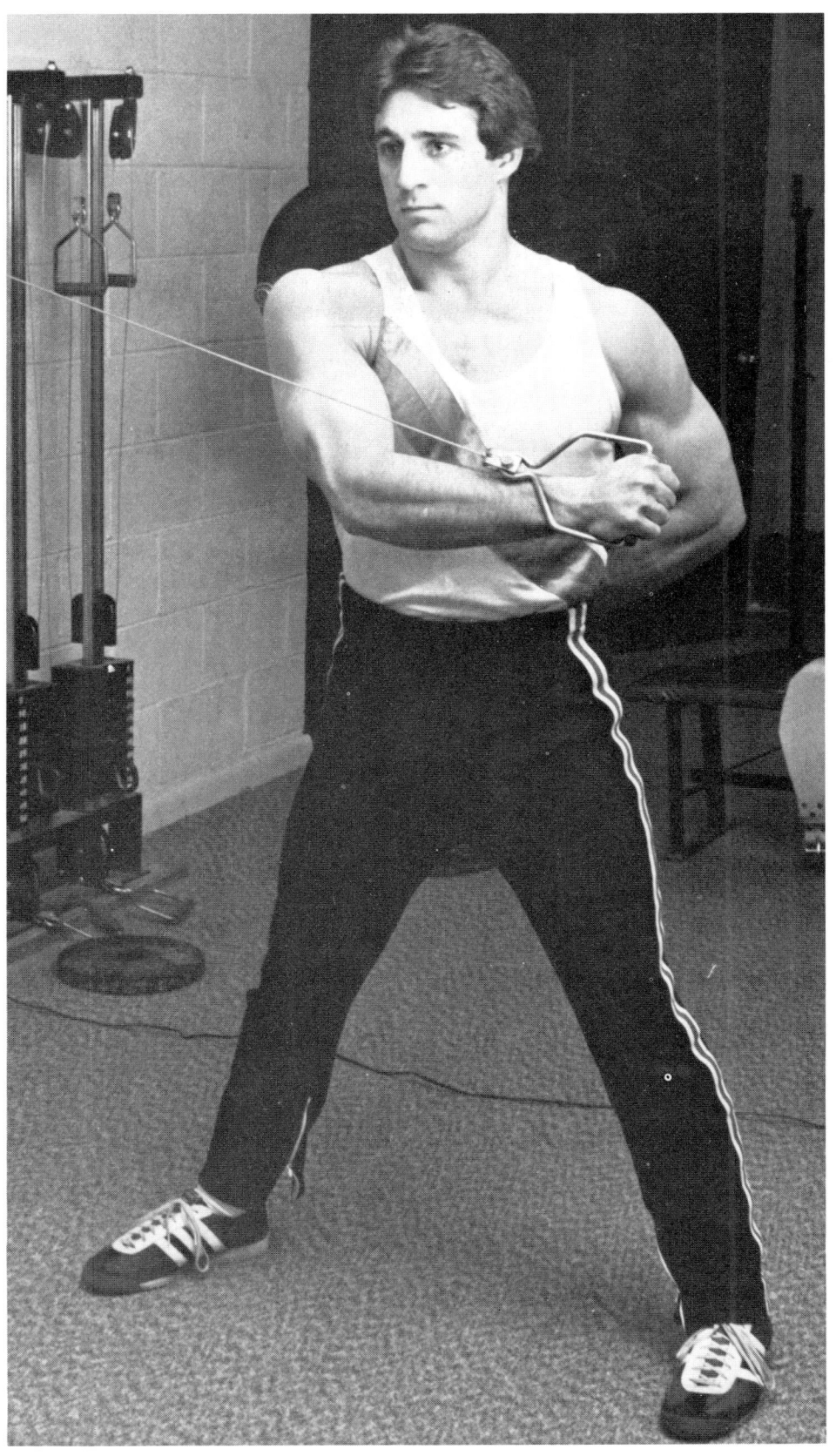

PULLS ACROSS THE chest with a cable apparatus are very effective for working the inner portions of the pectoral muscles.

THE "LAT MACHINE" is one of the most useful pieces of equipment found in health clubs. Pulling the bar down, as shown, develops the latissimus dorsi muscles, especially the upper parts.

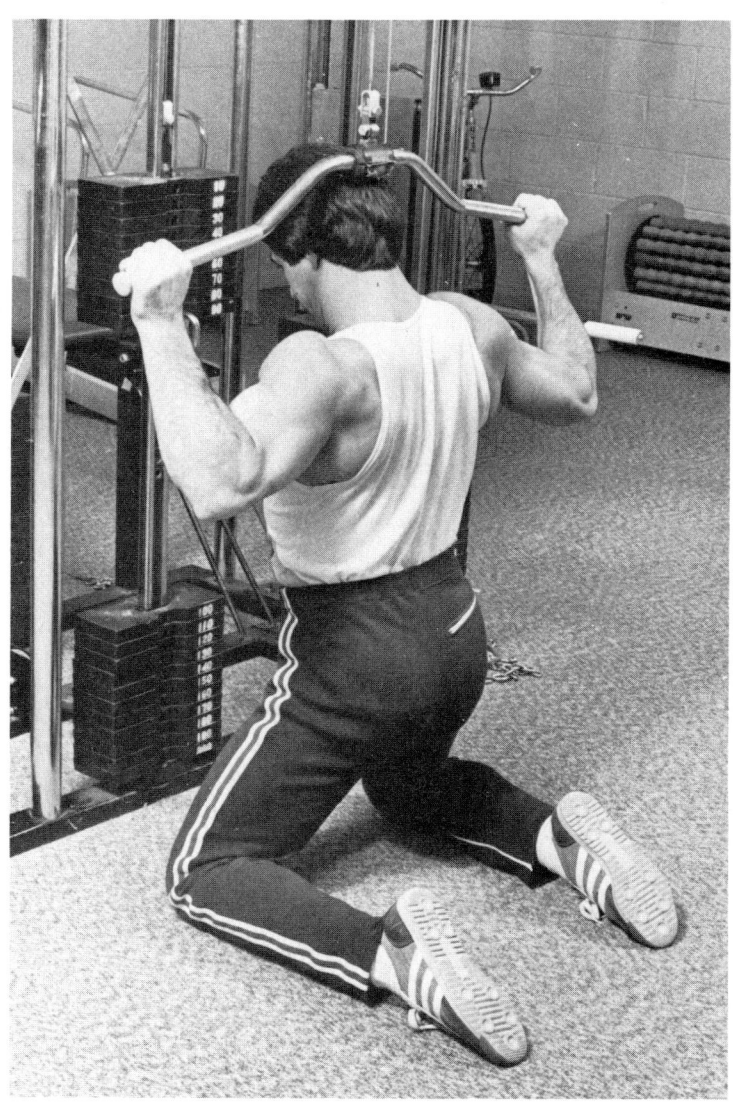

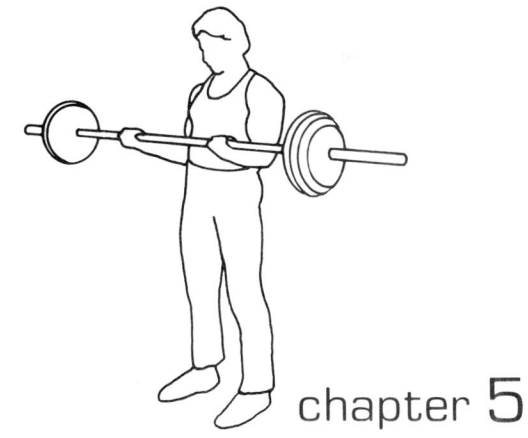

chapter 5

ORGANIZING BODYBUILDING ROUTINES

We now have covered basic bodybuilding exercises as well as more variation exercises than you would want to, or should, practice in a single workout. Let's consider how you might organize a training program for three hard workouts a week, starting with the key basic moves and adding additional movements where they are appropriate.

I. *Bench Press:* 10 + 8 + 6 + 4 + 2 with increasing weights and 10-15 reps, dropping back to the starting amount.
A. *Flying Exercise:* 3 sets of 10 reps.
a. *Incline Press:* 3 sets of 8-10 reps.
II. *Squat:* 10 + 8 + 6 + 4 + 2 with increasing weights.
A. *Front Squat:* 1–3 sets of 10–15 (light weight).
a. *OR Leg Curl:* 3 sets of 10; and *Leg Extension:* 3 sets of 10.
III. *Deep Breathing Pullover:* 10–15 reps, after last 3 sets of squats.

IV. *Rowing Exercise:* 3 sets of 8–12 reps.
A. *Bent-arm Pullover:* 3 sets of 8–10 reps.
a. *OR Lat Machine Pull-downs:* 3 sets of 10 reps.
B. *Stiff-legged Dead Lifts:* 3 sets of 10 reps.
a. *OR Hyperextension:* 3 sets of 10 reps.
V. *Sit-ups:* 20–50 reps, with or without weight, 1–3 sets.
A. *Twists:* with bar across shoulders, 40–100 reps.
a. *(Optional) Knee-ups or Leg-raises:* 10–50 reps.
VI. *Rise-on-Toes:* 3 sets of 10–20 reps.
A. *Seated Rise-on-Toes:* 3 sets of 10–20 reps.
a. *OR Donkey Raise:* 3 sets of 10–20 reps.
VII. *Barbell Curl:* 3 sets of 8–12 reps.
A. *Concentration Curl:* 3 sets of 10–12 reps.
a. *Preacher Bench Curl:* 3 sets of 10 reps.
B. *Triceps Extension:* standing or lying, 3 sets of 10 reps.

a. *Triceps Kick-backs:* 1–2 sets, 10 reps.
b. *OR Triceps Push-down:* 2–3 sets, 10 reps.
VIII. *Barbell (or Two Dumbbells) Press:* 3 sets of 8–12 reps.
A. *Lateral Raise:* 3 sets of 10 reps.
a. *Lateral Raise, Leaning:* 3 sets of 10 reps.

GETTING INTO A ROUTINE

The foregoing is a tough bodybuilding workout, and it would take a real workhorse to complete it. It assumes that you have about two hours of time available to exercise and that you are going to move along without long rest breaks between sets and exercises. It is definitely not a workout that you would jump right into.

The way to work into a routine such as this one is to perform all the basic exercises (those marked with Roman numerals) and add one set at a time of the first variation movements listed (those with capital letters). You may not want to go to the third level (small letters), or you may not be able to since some of them call for special equipment. But if you do, add them a set at a time until you become accustomed to the full routine.

This three-tiered workout also assumes that you have no special problems, no areas of your body that need more work than others. If you do have special problem areas, work to the third tier with exercises for those parts, and only do the first or second tier of exercises where your body is already well developed and well shaped.

As mentioned earlier, you may not want to work as intensively on bench presses and squats as this routine requires. In that case, do one light set of ten reps as a warm-up in each exercise, and then do three sets of eight to twelve reps with a weight that feels right for that many repetitions. No two people are alike, and you must learn to experiment with exercises, sets, and reps until you find the combination that works best for you. The object is to set up a routine that not only includes exercises for the major muscle groups of the body but also gets you into the habit of taking an all-around workout that does not neglect any body part. By including at least one exercise, and sufficient sets, for every major muscle group, you will not develop a lopsided, out-of-balance physique.

Importance of Sequence

Notice the sequence of exercises, putting the heaviest movements—bench press and squat—at the beginning of the basic movements in order to handle heavy weights in these growth-promoters. Additional chest exercises are inserted after the bench press to enhance the pump of blood to the chest muscles, and lighter leg exercises follow the heavy squats for the same reason. Then come the exercises, both basic and variation movements, that work the back, midsection, calves, arms, and shoulders.

Many bodybuilders will do abdominal exercises first, both to "get them out of the way" and to use them as a general warm-up. That is a good approach, but in a full-body routine, to be done three days a week, shifting to exercises for the midsection and calves midway through allows your arms and shoulders an opportunity to recover from their participation in the chest and back exercises. Most young male bodybuilders like the feeling of pumped arms and shoulders, which continues for awhile after a workout in which these body parts are exercised last.

SPLIT ROUTINES

An alternative to a workout in which all body parts are exercised during the same training session is the so-called split routine. Such a routine would take the same exercises, but break them up so that you work chest, back, and shoulders on, say, Mondays, Wednesdays, and Fridays and abdominals, thighs, calves, and arms on Tuesdays, Thursdays, and Saturdays. Once you are conditioned to the split routine, you will find that it permits you to increase the amount of work in each exercise (more sets, more weight, an additional variation, or any combination of these elements). These increases are possible because it does not take as much time and energy to do half of the divided workout in each session.

Staying with the same basic approach we have been considering, here is how the exercises can be divided into a split routine.

Monday-Wednesday-Friday

I. *Bench Press:* 10 + 8 + 6 + 4 + 2 with increasing weights and 10–15 reps, dropping back to the starting amount. (Or warm-up set of 10 followed by 3–5 sets of 8–12.)
A. *Flying Exercise:* 3–5 sets of 10 reps.
a. *Incline Press:* 3–5 sets of 8–10 reps.
II. *Rowing Exercise:* 3–5 sets of 8–12 reps.
A. *Bent-arm Pullover:* 3–5 sets of 8–10 reps.

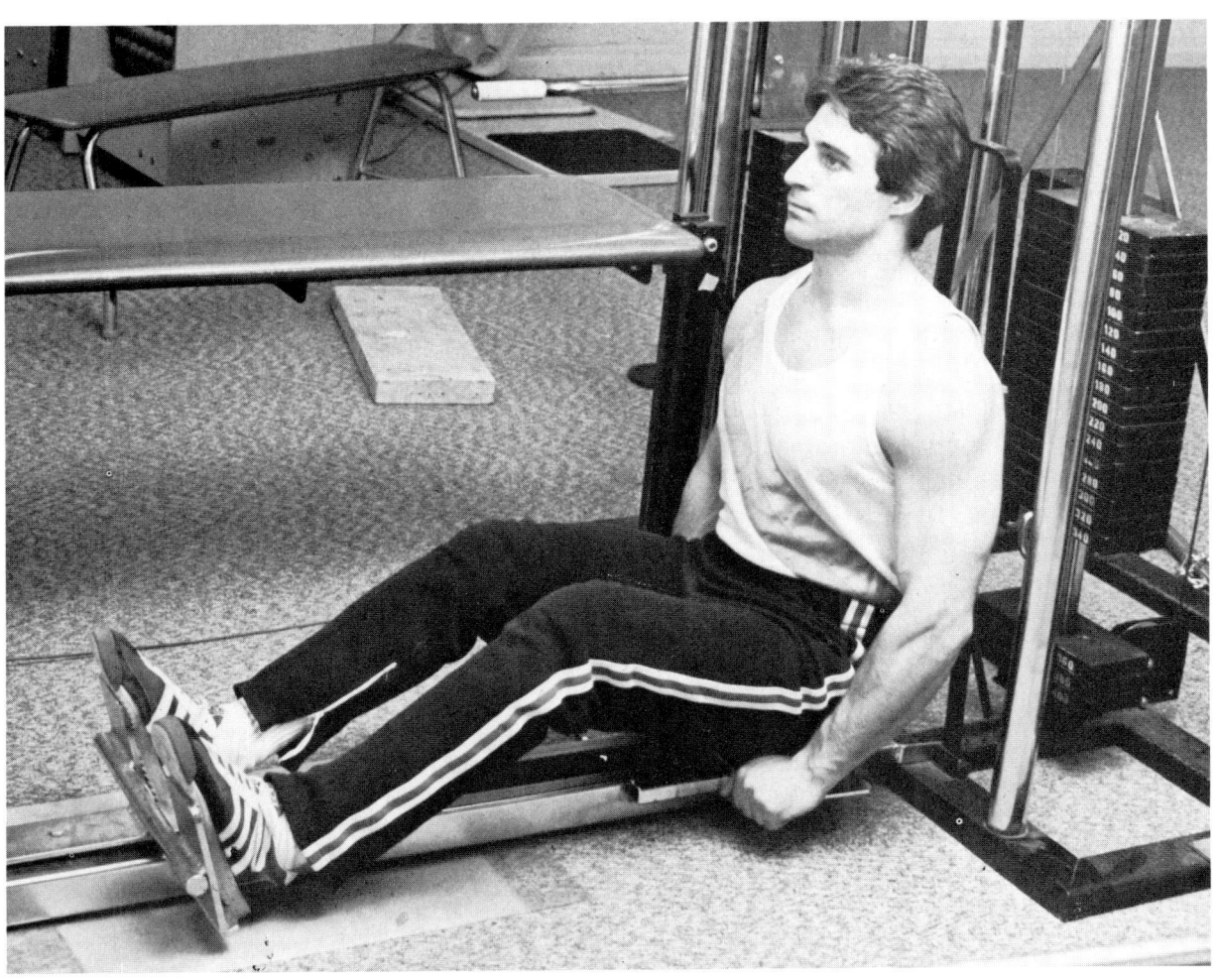

A LEG PRESS MACHINE makes it possible to exercise the thigh muscles against very heavy resistance.

a.*Chins:* wide and narrow grip, 3–6 sets.
OR Lat Machine Pull-downs: 3–5 sets.
B.*Stiff-legged Dead Lifts:* 3 sets of 10 reps.
Or Hyperextension: 3 sets of 10 reps.
   III.*Barbell (or Two Dumbbells) Press:* 3–5 sets of 8–10 reps.
A.*Lateral Raise:* 3–5 sets of 10 reps.
a.*Lateral Raise, Leaning:* 3–5 sets of 10 reps.

The foregoing Monday-Wednesday-Friday routine focuses on exercises for the chest, back (upper and lower), and shoulders. Note that sets are given as 3–5 (meaning three to five). You should appraise your own needs objectively and do five sets for the body parts most lacking in development, three where no catch-up is needed. Most competitive bodybuilders preparing for contests do five or more sets for all body parts.

The following program includes the second part of the split routine, working the midsection, thighs, calves, and arms. (Many bodybuilders do exercises for the midsection during every workout, and almost as many include calf exercises during every workout.)

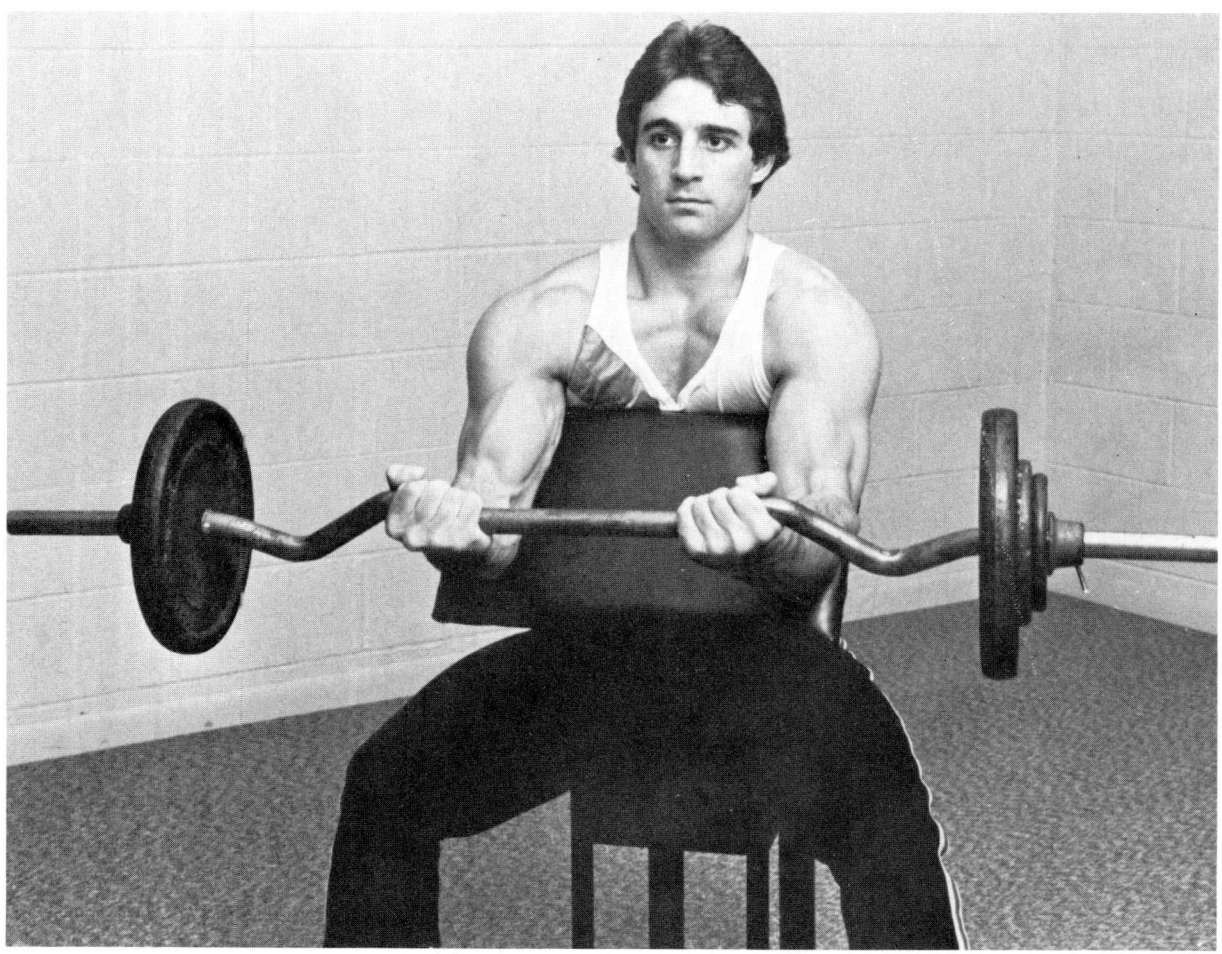

THE "PREACHER BENCH," which looks like a reversed lectern, is an especially good piece of apparatus for isolating and focusing work on the biceps. The bent "curl bar" helps, too, but the exercise can be done with a straight bar or a pair of dumbbells.

Tuesday-Thursday-Saturday

IV. *Sit-ups:* 3–5 sets of 20–50 reps.
A. *Twists:* 1–3 sets of 40–100 reps.
a. *Knee-ups OR Leg-raises:* 1–3 sets of 20–50 reps.
V. *Squat:* 10 + 8 + 6 + 4 + 2 with increasing weights.
A. *Front Squat:* 3–5 sets of 10–15 (light weight).
a. *Leg Curl:* 3–5 sets of 10, AND
b. *Leg Extension:* 3–5 sets of 10.
c. *(Optional) Leg Presses:* 3–5 sets of 10–15.
VI. *Deep Breathing Pullover:* 10–15 reps after last 3–5 sets of squats.
VII. *Rise-on-Toes:* 5–8 sets of 10–20 reps.
A. *Seated Rise-on-Toes:* 3–5 sets of 10–20 reps.
a. *Donkey Raise:* 3–5 sets of 10–20 reps.
VIII. *Barbell (or Two Dumbbells) Curl:* 5 sets of 8–12 reps.
A. *Concentration Curl:* 3–5 sets of 10–12 reps.

a. *Preacher Bench Curl:* 3 sets of 10 reps.
b. *Wrist Curl:* (palms up and down) 6 sets of 10–15 reps.
B. *Triceps Extension, Supine:* 5 sets of 8–12 reps.
a. *Triceps Extension, Standing:* 3–5 sets of 8–12 reps.
b. *OR Triceps Push-down:* 3–5 sets of 8–12 reps.
c. *Triceps Kick-backs:* 3–5 sets of 10 reps.

The split routine still provides all the basic exercises, but it provides more flexibility for concentration of effort. The third tier becomes more or less optional, but wrist curls should be added to an arm portion of a split routine since no one training at this intensity should neglect some direct work for every body part. The forearms do obtain benefit from holding onto the bar in many exercises, but advanced bodybuilders need specialized forearm work.

THE EXCEPTIONAL MUSCULAR DEVELOPMENT and fine proportions that won Mr. America and Mr. Universe titles for Boyer Coe are evident in this picture, taken during a posing exhibition.

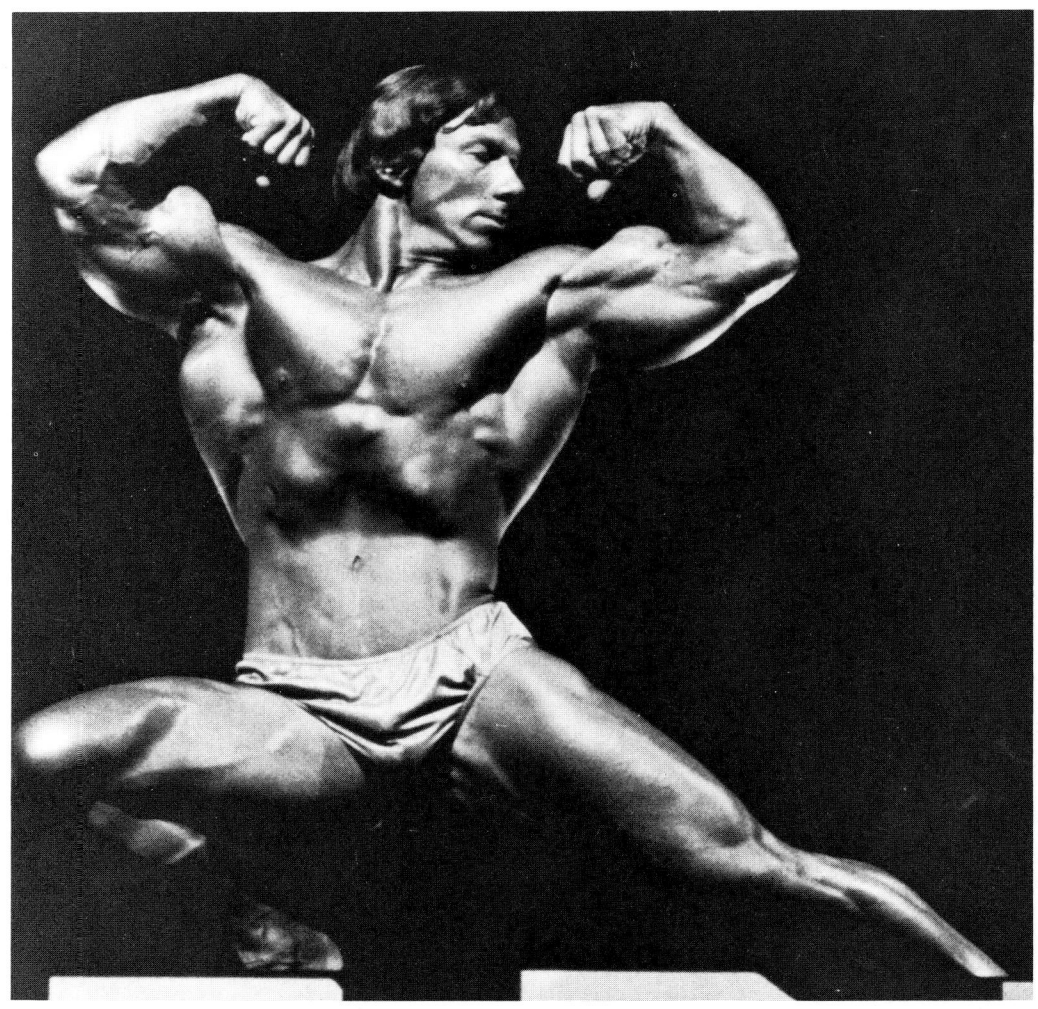

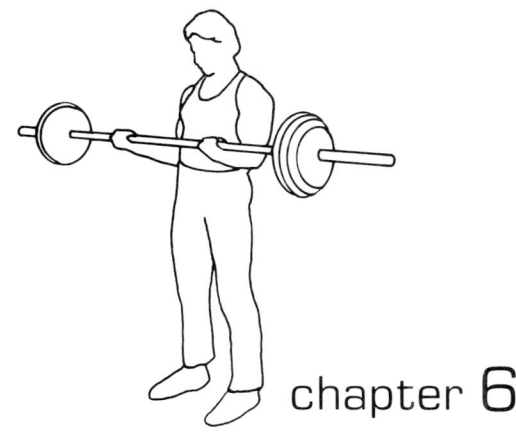

chapter 6

TRAINING TO BECOME MR. UNIVERSE

The evolution of a training program from advanced to super-advanced can be illustrated by two routines followed by Boyer Coe. The first one led to major prominence as Teen-age Mr. America of 1966. The second routine was used in 1977 to improve the muscular development that had won him Mr. America and the international Mr. Universe titles in 1969.

THE 1966 ROUTINE

Bear in mind that Coe was already an advanced bodybuilder when he won the teen-age title, having previously won the Mr. Southern U.S.A., Mr. Louisiana, and other major contests against experienced men in events with no age restrictions. Under the guidance of Lloyd "Red" Lerille, a capable instructor who was himself a Mr. America winner in 1960, Coe was following this six-days-a-week split routine:

Monday and Thursday

Exercise	Sets	Reps
Bench Press	4	6
Inclined Bench Press	4	8
Dips	4	8
Press Behind Neck	4	6
Press on Press Machine	4	8
Lateral Raises	4	8
Push-down on Lat Machine	4	8
Triceps Extension on Bench	4	8
Reverse Grip Triceps Extension on Bench	4	8

Tuesday and Friday

Exercise	Sets	Reps
Squat (full)	4	6
Leg Press	4	8
Leg Extension	4	8
Chins (back of neck)	4	8
Chins (front, wide grip)	4	8
Pull-Down on Lat Machine	4	8
Incline Bench Curl	4	8
Curl on Preacher Bench	4	8
Regular Curl	4	8

Wednesday and Saturday

Exercise	Sets	Reps
High Pulls	4	6
Shoulder Shrug (barbell)	4	8
Shoulder Shrug (dumbbells)	4	8
Stiff-Legged Dead Lift	4	8
Prone Hyperextensions	4	10
Forearm Work	10	20

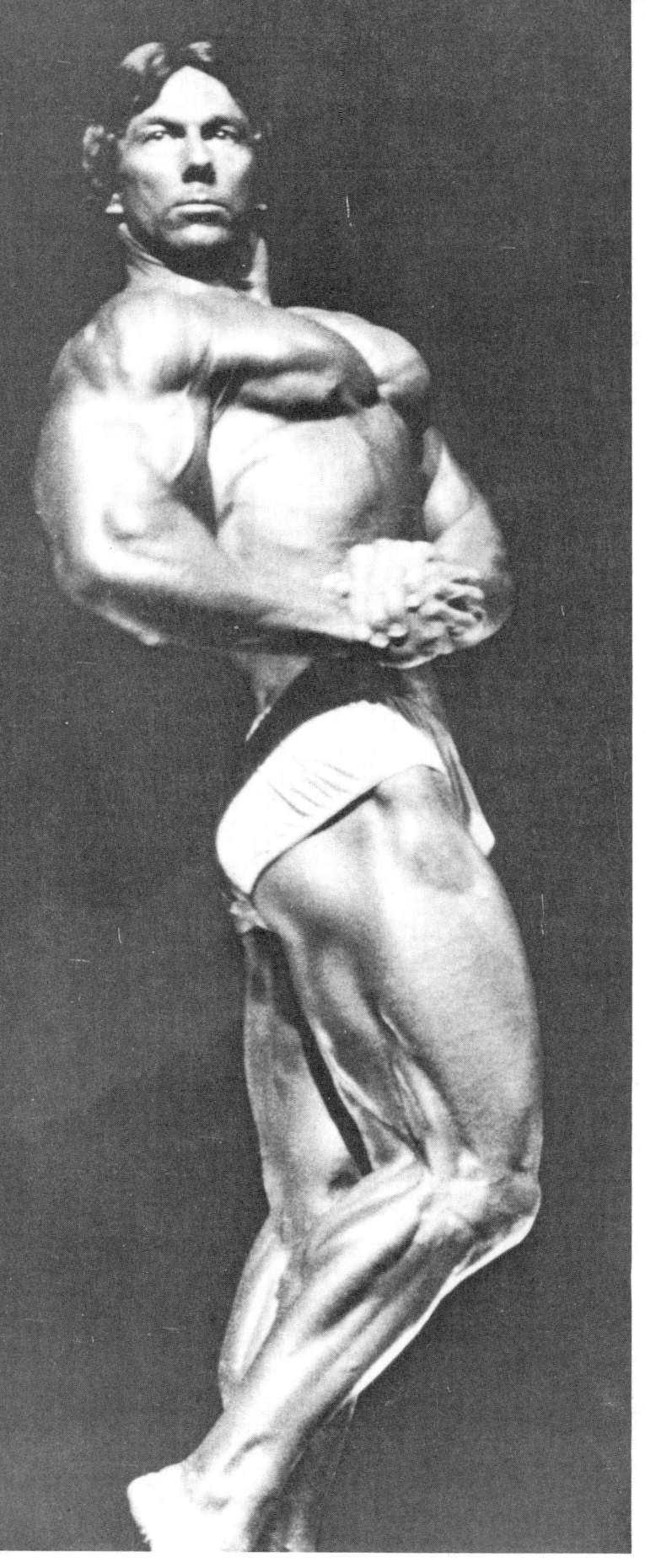

UNDER TENSION, Boyer Coe's chest muscles show a clear-cut line of definition between the upper and lower sections of pectoral. Note also the unusual thigh biceps and calf development, often lacking in even top-flight bodybuilders.

In the foregoing routine, Coe concentrated on chest, shoulders, and triceps on Mondays and Thursdays; he worked thighs, back, and triceps on Tuesdays and Fridays; and he worked trapezius and low back on Wednesdays and Saturdays. He worked his abdominal muscles and calves during every workout, Monday through Saturday, doing sit-ups, leg-raises, and twists, plus the basic rise-on-toes exercise. At a time, Coe also was competing as a power lifter, and he placed second in the Southwestern Championships, 198-pound class, with a squat of 465, bench press of 355, and dead lift of 500 pounds.

GAINING NATIONAL PROMINENCE

It took Boyer Coe approximately four years to reach the point where he became a contender on the national scene. He had begun bodybuilding at 15 and, by a combination of natural aptitude, determination, and hard work, had won the Mr. New Orleans title at 17, the day before he graduated from high school. He suffered disappointments, too, losing the Teen-Age Mr. America title to Dennis Tinerino (who later also won Mr. America) before winning it the following year. He lost the 1968 Mr. America title to broad-shouldered Jim Haislop, then won in 1969 and turned the tables on Haislop by beating him in the Mr. Universe contest in London.

A friendly, helpful person, it was only natural for Boyer Coe to become interested in the gym business. What better way could he make use of the great fund of knowledge about exercise and nutrition that he had accumulated from his own experience and his association with other top men in the field? He opened Boyer Coe's Body-Masters gym, which he equipped with both standard bodybuilding apparatus and special, customized equipment that he found especially helpful in advanced training.

Whereas Coe initially trained for both power lifting and bodybuilding, he no longer does the power lifts. (Before abandoning that sport, however, he had registered best lifts of 500 squat, 420 bench press, and 550 dead lift early in his career.) Now he carefully analyzes his body and employs only those exercises that he feels will best improve his proportions, concentrating on movements that overcome what he perceives as weaknesses (a less discerning eye would have difficulty finding any!) and eliminating exercises that he feels might overdevelop one body part in relation to another. For example, he stopped doing heavy, regular barbell bench presses because he found they developed too much anterior deltoid muscle and produced an imbalance in his physique.

THE 1977 ROUTINE

Coe's advanced program in 1977 consisted of a mixture of standard bodybuilding moves and special exercises, making use of customized equipment. The program follows (with illustrations showing some of the innovative variations and special equipment):

Monday and Wednesday

Midsection: Twists
Sit-ups on steep incline
Hanging Knee-ups

Calves: Rise-on-Toes on curved-seat leg press machine
Regular Rise-on-Toes

Shoulders: Press Behind Neck, Seated
Lateral Raises, Leaning
Rear deltoid machine

Chest: Incline Bench Press
Flying Exercise (vertical machine)
Bench Press (vertical machine)
Iron cross machine
Dumbbell Pullovers

Triceps: Lat Machine Push-downs (close grip)
Supine Triceps Extension, dumbbells
Triceps Extension, Leaning
Kick-backs (or triceps machine exercise)
One-arm Triceps extensions

Tuesday and Thursday

Midsection: Same as Monday and Wednesday

Calves: Same as Monday and Wednesday

Thighs: Back Squats on "Power Driver"
Front Squats on "Power Driver"
Leg Extension
Leg Curl

Back: Chins behind neck
Low pulley rowing
Close-grip lat pulls
Low pulley rowing
Shrugs with dumbbells
Low back machine

Biceps: Preacher Bench Curls
Dumbbell Curls on incline
Preacher Bench Curls with dumbbells
Reverse Curls

Coe starts his workouts by doing 200 seated twists, both to increase the muscularity of the sides of his waist and to warm up his low back. After the twists, he supersets all his exercises, beginning with hanging knee-ups (see photo) and sit-ups on a high board with a 40-pound weight held behind his head. In the knee-ups, his performance is very strict, going from full hang to a point where his knees touch his chest for ten sets of fifteen reps. The sit-ups that he alternates with knee-ups are done as a muscle-building exercise in sets of ten, the weight and leverage of the incline intensifying the effect on the abdominal muscles.

The calf exercises also are supersetted, a set of twenty calf pushes on the leg press machine and a set of the regular rise-on-toes, also twenty reps, for a total

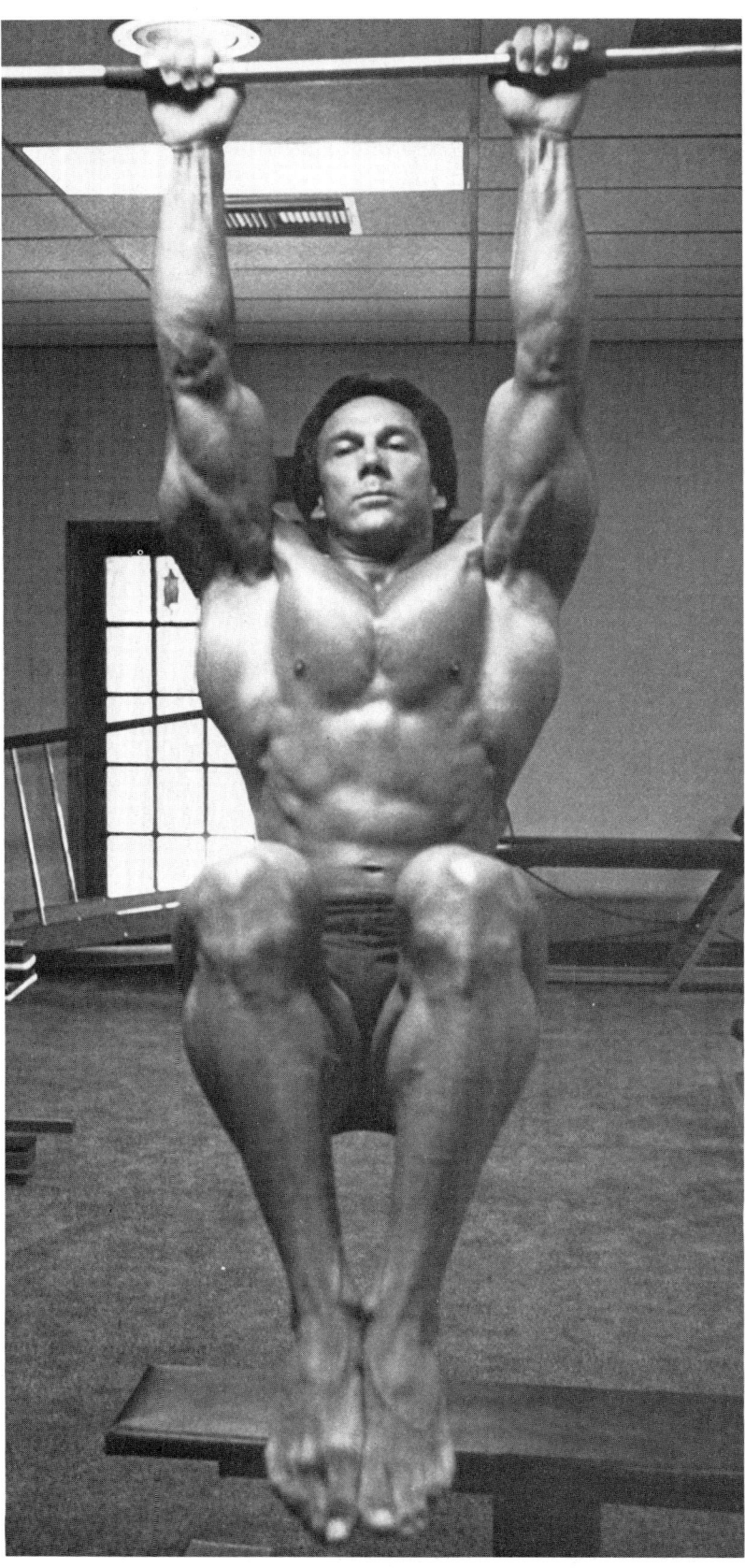

BOYER COE does knee-ups from a hanging position. He considers this the best exercise for the lower abdominal muscles.

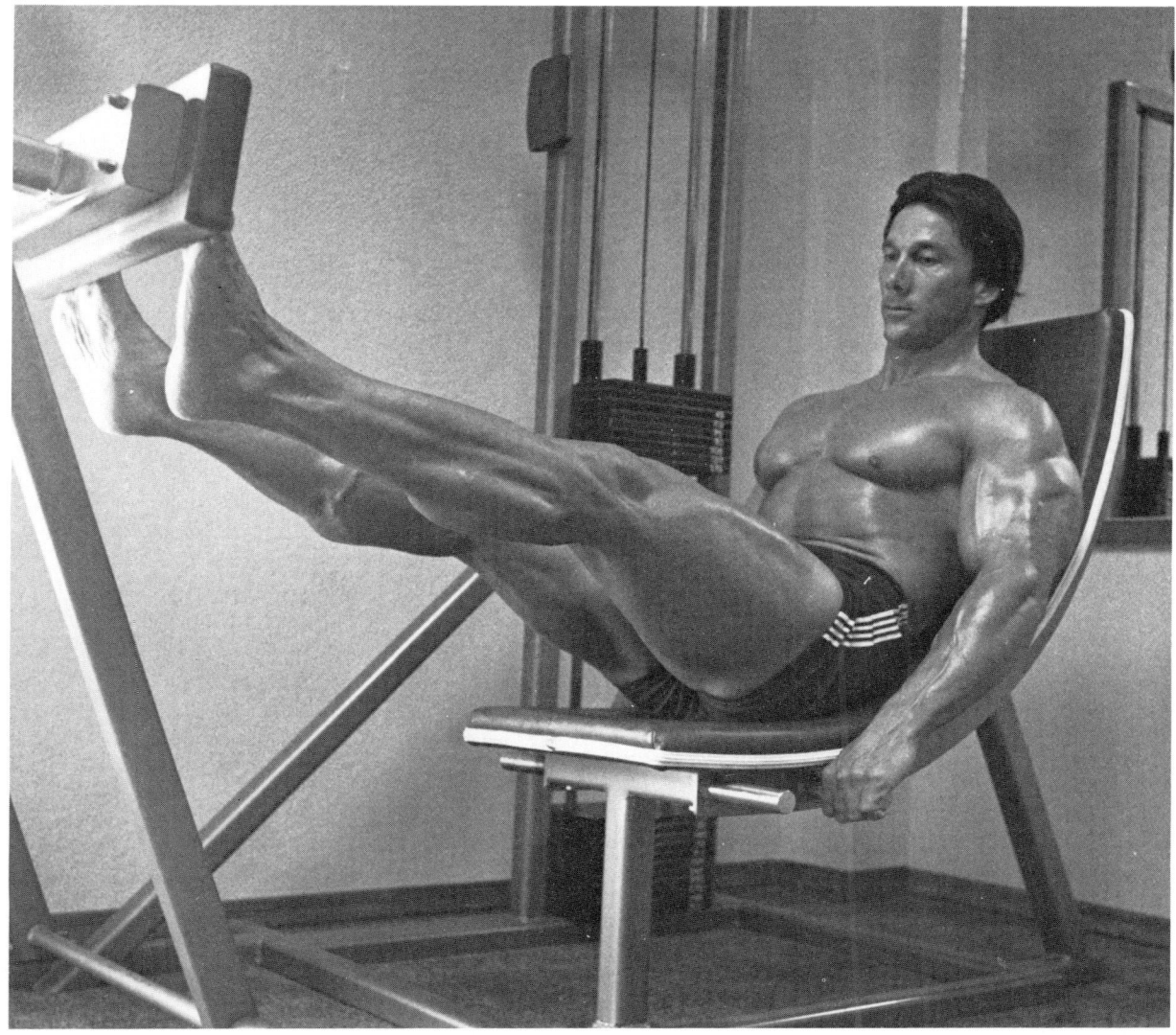

A SPECIAL LEG PRESS MACHINE is used by Coe for part of his calf-developing routine.

of ten sets of each exercise. Both the abdominal and calf exercises are done on four successive days, Monday through Thursday.

Coe believes that it is important to stretch the calf muscles thoroughly in the rise-on-toes exercise and recommends that the block under the toes be high enough to provide a complete stretching action.

The Monday and Wednesday Workout

On Mondays and Wednesdays, Coe pro-

ceeds to a series of shoulder exercises, including the lateral raise, use of a rear deltoid machine that provides an action similar to the leaning lateral raise, and barbell presses behind neck, seated. His lateral raise is a special variation in which he attaches a strong belt to the wall behind him so he can lean forward slightly as he raises the dumbbells, concentrating on keeping a slight forward tilt of the dumbbell handles. The lean and the hand position combine to focus the work on the lateral (side) head of the deltoid. The

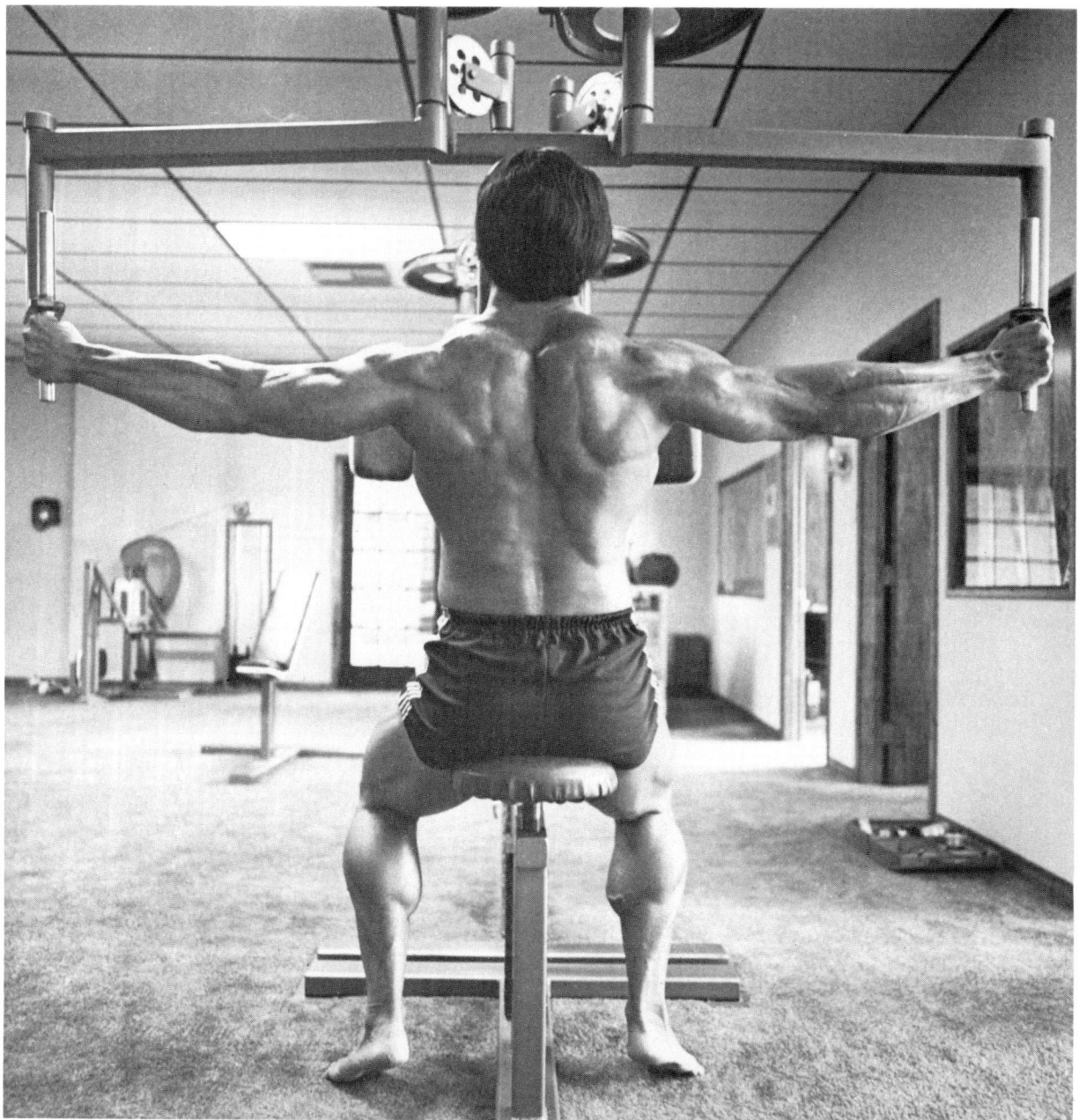

A SPECIAL REAR DELTOID MACHINE enables Coe to concentrate on the back portions of his shoulders as he pulls the handles backward.

rear deltoid machine focuses the work on the back portion of the deltoid, and the presses work both the anterior (front) and lateral heads.

Coe also incorporates other exercises for the deltoids from time to time, to work his shoulders from all angles. He does a total of thirty sets of shoulder exercises, about ten reps per set. In the seated press, he does five sets, concentrating on handling as much weight as he can in strict form.

In his chest routine, Coes devotes a lot of time to the upper part of the pectorals

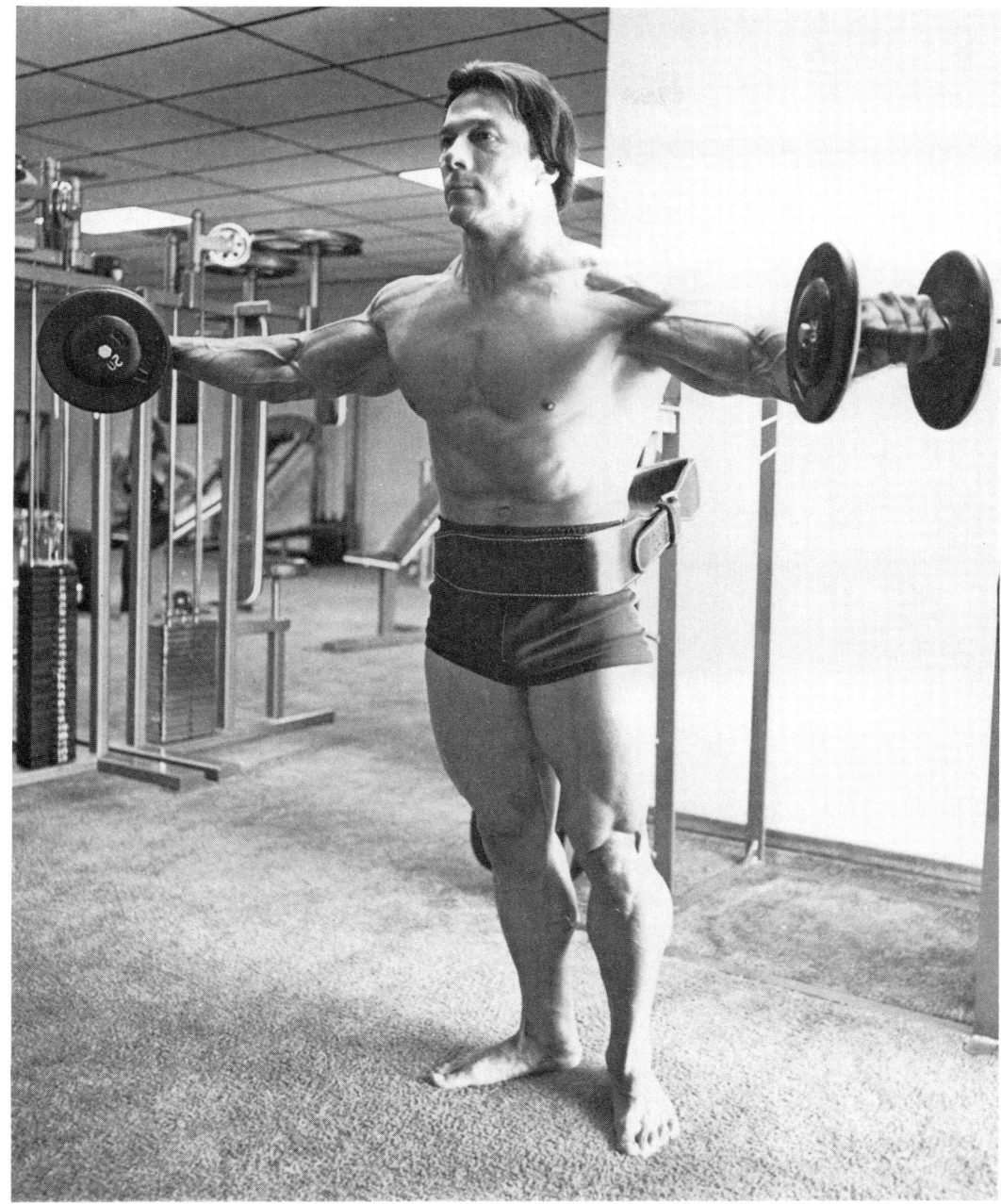

BY LEANING INTO A BELT that is attached to the wall behind him and by keeping the dumbbells level, Coe individualizes the lateral raise in order to isolate the sides of his deltoids. Note how the lateral portion stands out as he raises the weights.

because this portion is hard to develop. He uses incline presses with a barbell, touching the barbell to the base of his neck to get a good stretch. He does the flying exercise, using a machine that allows him to work in the vertical position rather than lying on a bench and using dumbbells. The machine also provides resistance at the completion of the movement, which fully develops the inner portion of the pectorals where they attach at the sternum. He does bench presses on a

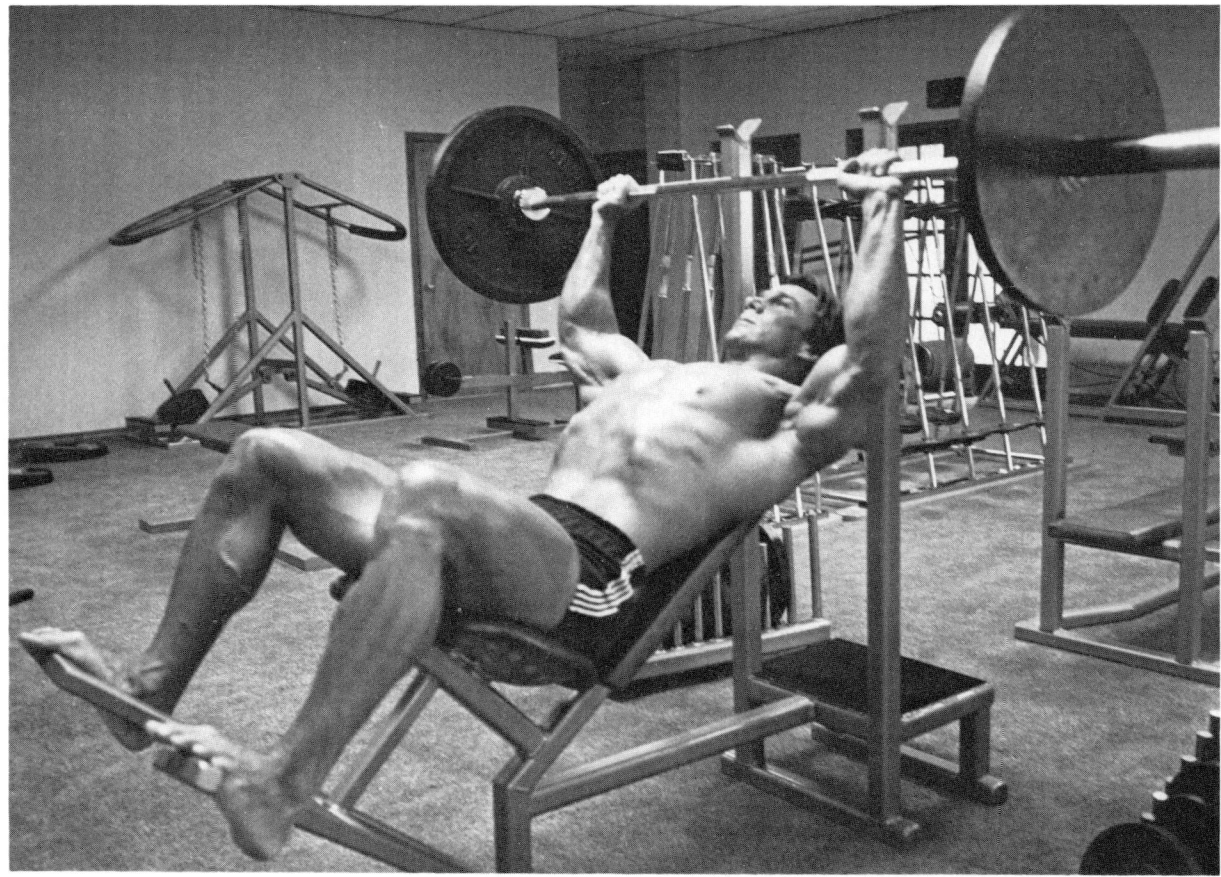

THE INCLINE PRESS WITH BARBELL is Coe's favorite exercise for the upper part of the pectoral muscles.

vertical machine rather than with a barbell (see illustration) and pullovers with a dumbbell to stretch the rib cage. Coe also has another special machine, similar to the apparatus used for the flying exercise, for focused pectoral contractions.

The final body part that Coe exercises on Mondays and Wednesdays is the triceps. First, he supersets triceps pushdowns (close grip) on the lat machine with the over head triceps extension (seated). These first two exercises, practiced alternately (about ten reps of one, followed by ten reps of the other), are intended to produce mass in the big muscle at the back of the arm. Then he supersets triceps extensions with dumbbells (seated on an incline bench) with triceps kick-backs for density and definition.

Sometimes he substitutes work on a triceps machine for kick-backs, and he may also do one-arm triceps extensions.

Counting all the sets, Coe does from twenty to thirty sets for each body part, which results in each muscle performing from two hundred to three hundred contractions and extensions in a workout.

The Tuesday and Thursday Workout

On Tuesdays and Thursdays, Boyer Coe starts with the same abdominal and calf exercises that he does on Mondays and Wednesdays. Then he moves on to exercises for his thighs, supersetting front and back squats on an angled "Power Driver" machine. He warms up with a light set of twenty reps and then works with heavier

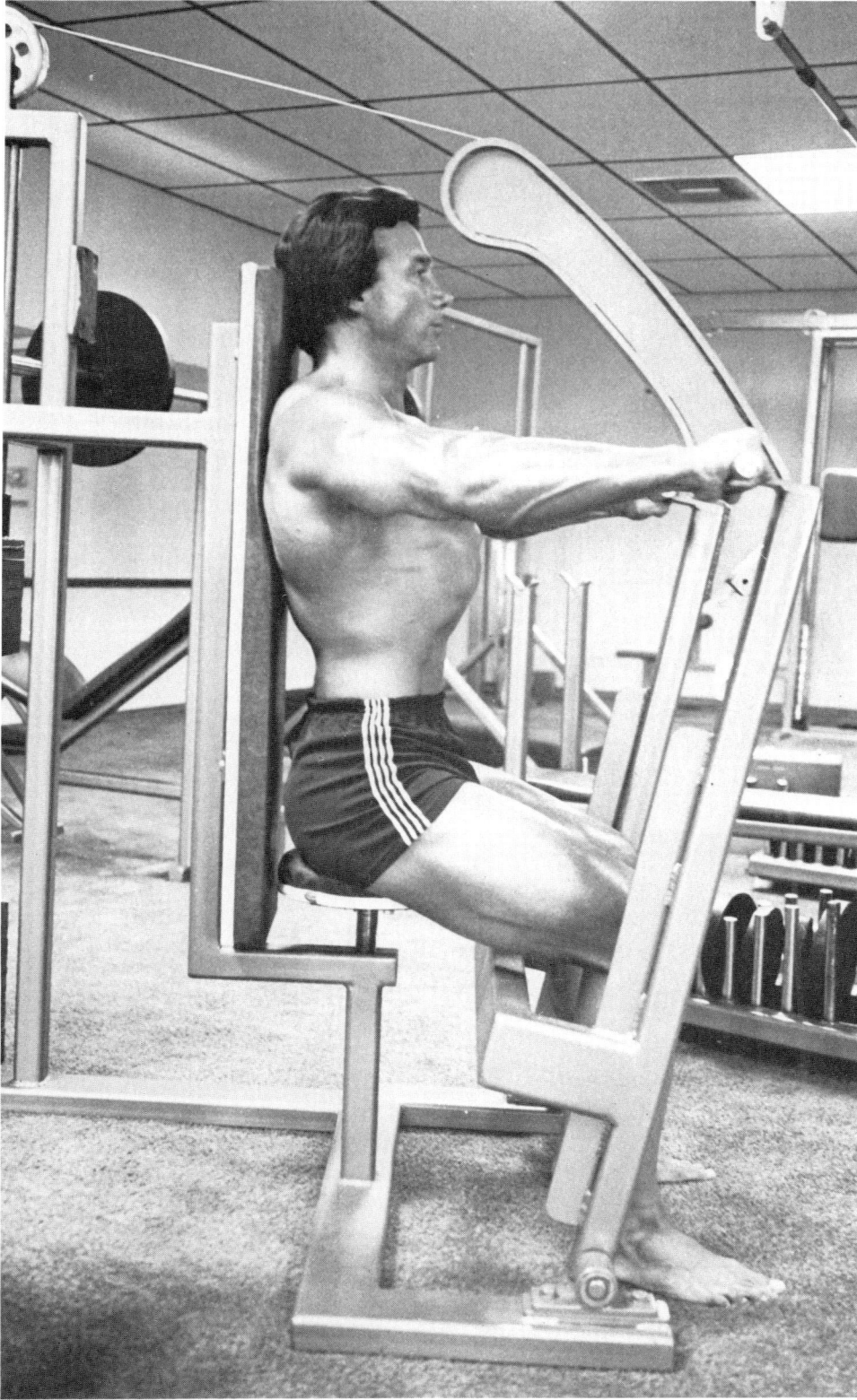

THIS SPECIAL APPARATUS allows Coe to perform a slightly varied bench press movement while seated upright.

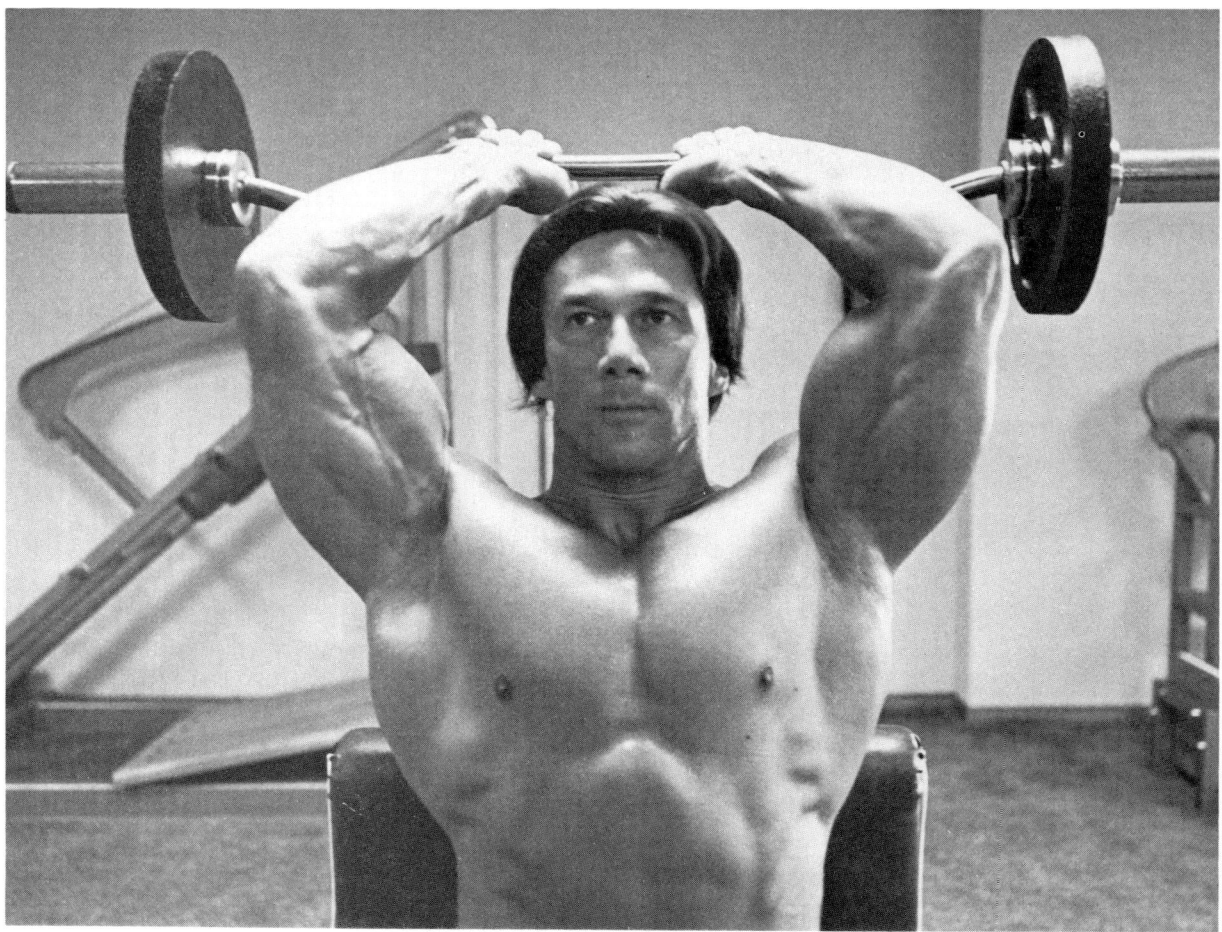

COE SUPERSETS TRICEPS EXTENSIONS with lat machine push-downs to build muscle mass at the back of the arms.

weights, concentrating on getting as low as possible to fully stretch the muscles, but also being careful to keep a flat back and focus the work on his thighs, not on his hips and/or back. Coe does seven sets in each position. Then he supersets leg extensions and leg curls. He feels that a fully-developed thigh biceps is very important to a physique contestant and works very hard on the leg curls.

Coe works his back hard and from many angles, beginning by supersetting chins (varying the hand-spacing from wide to narrow) with low cable rowing. Then he moves on to a tri-set of pulley rowing (again) with lat machine pull-downs and shrugs while holding two

dumbbells. In other words, he does a set of pulley rows, a set of lat pulls, and a set of shrugs; then he starts around again. Finally, he works his low back with a special machine in which he applies resistance from a strap across the back of his neck, leaning well forward as though doing a good-morning exercise or stiff-legged dead lift, and completes the movement with a hyperextension (see illustration). The weight used is in a stack attached to a pulley, which runs around a cam to supply high intensity resistance through the full range of motion. Coe does six sets of fifteen reps in this special low-back exercise.

Finally, Coe works his biceps by super-

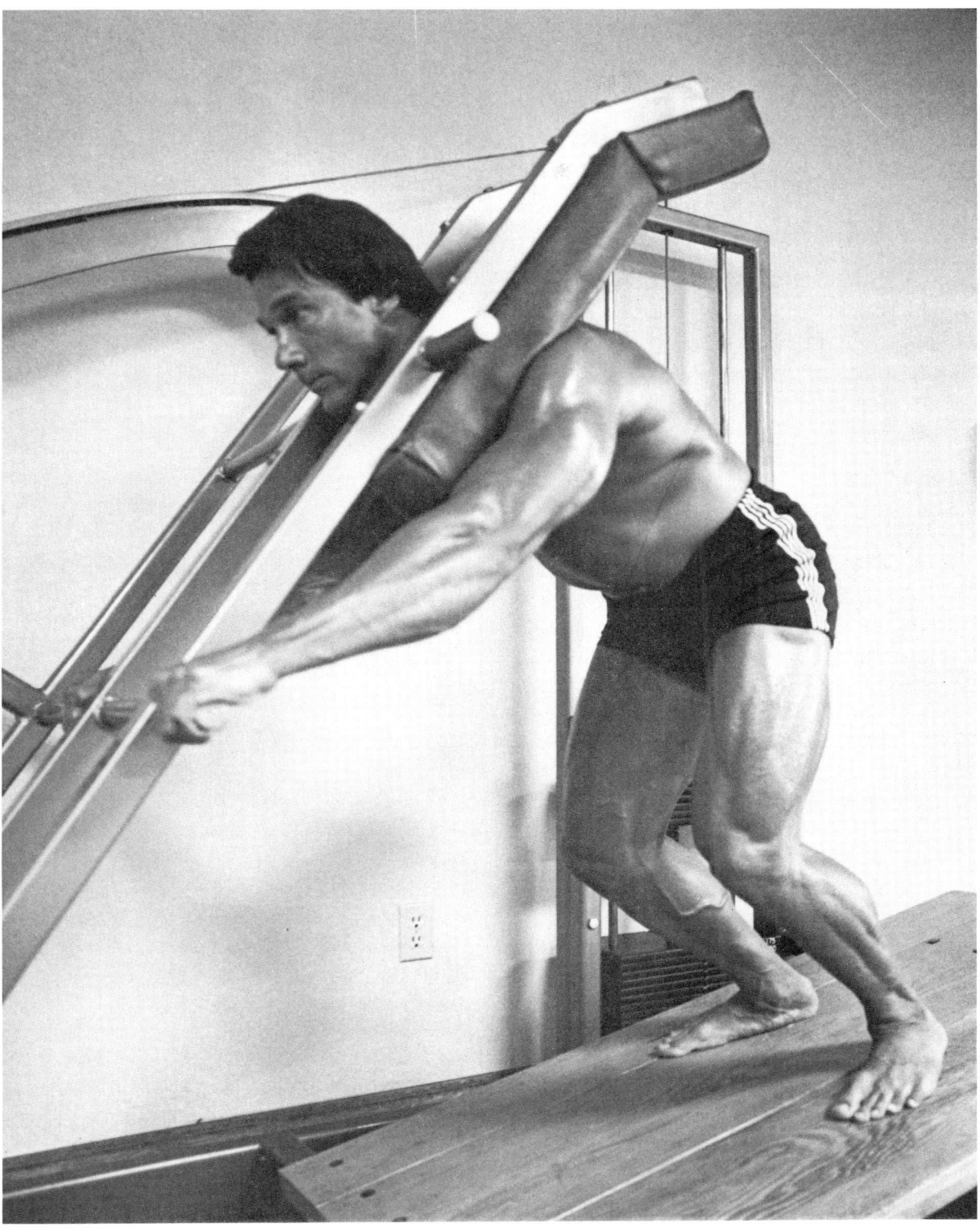

FRONT SQUATS on a "Power Driver" machine work Coe's thighs much as a football charging sled would, except that he moves deliberately, focusing on thigh muscle action.

BACK SQUATS on the "Power Driver" are done leaning backward to concentrate on thigh development, much as the old-fashioned "Hack squat" does. (In the Hack squat, a weight is held behind the hips.)

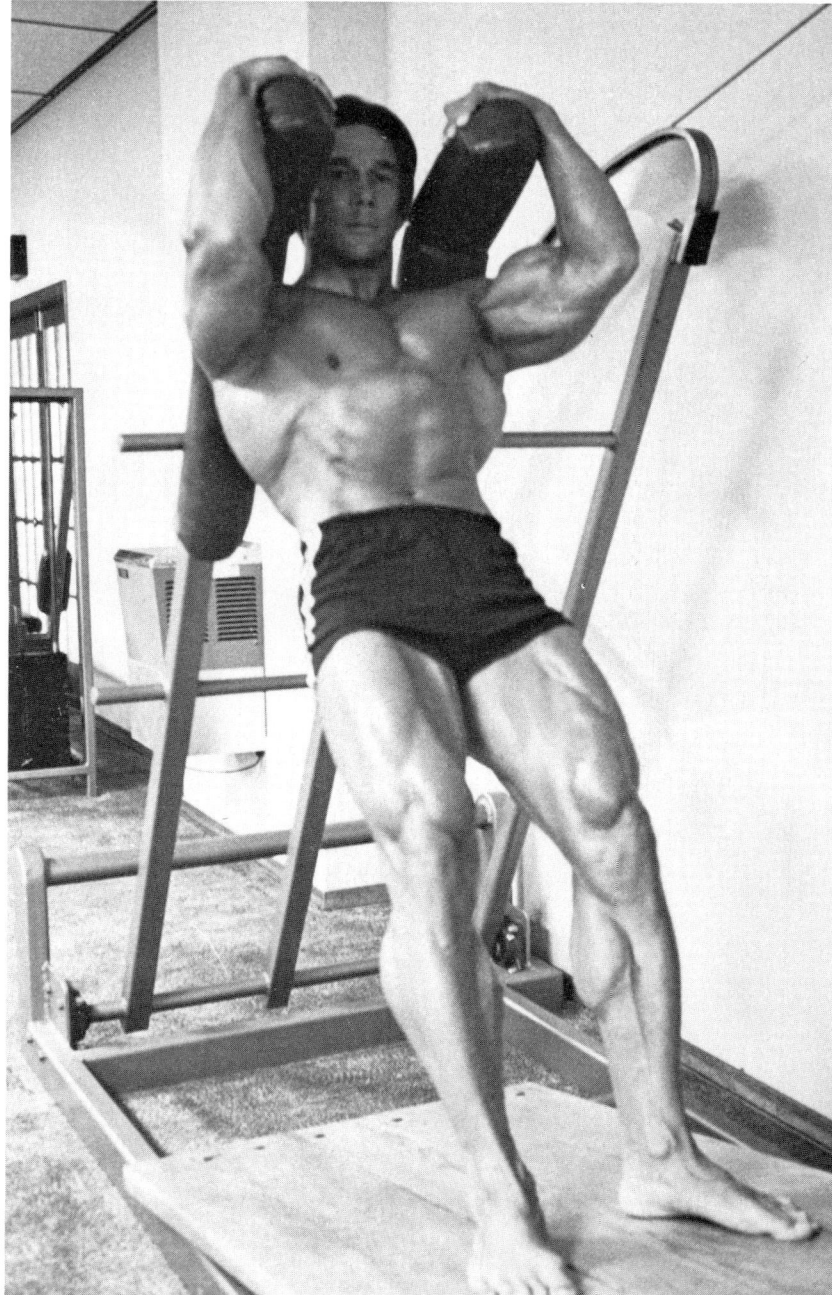

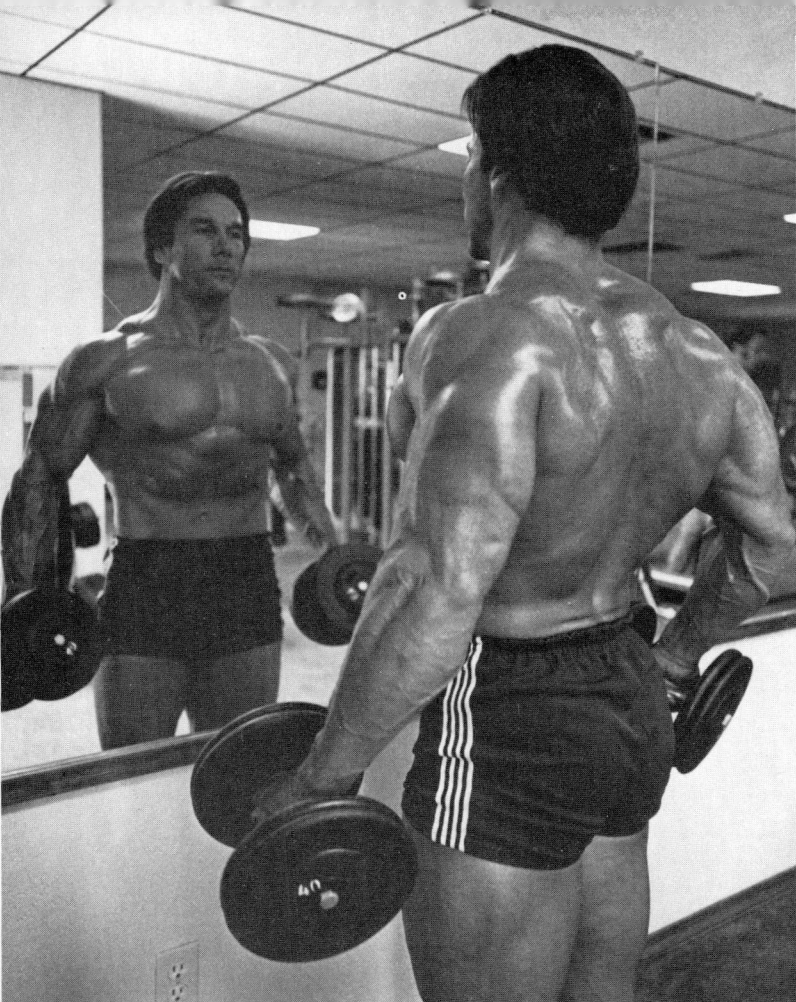

SHRUGS WITH TWO DUMBBELLS, in which he tries to raise his shoulders as close to his ears as possible, is Coe's favorite method for developing the trapezius muscle that runs between the neck and the deltoids.

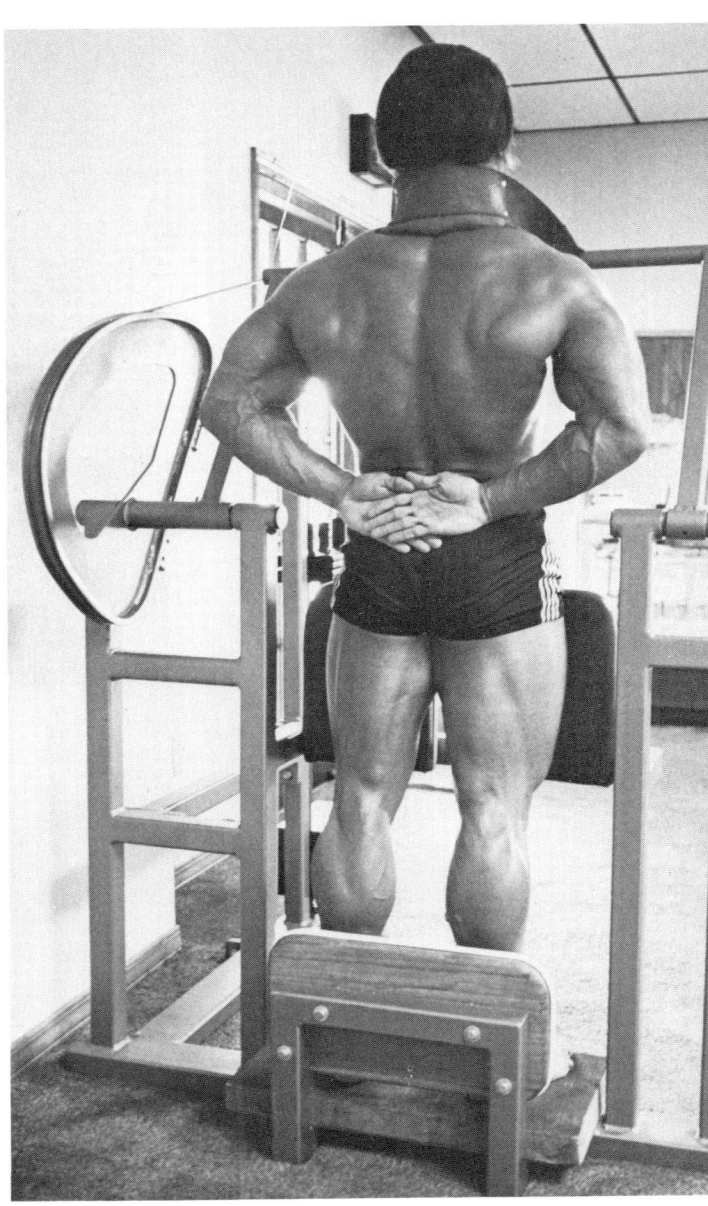

THE SPECIAL APPARATUS shown enables Coe to stretch and contract his low back muscles over a full range of motion. Note that he is braced at the front of his thighs so he can lean well forward as well as back against the resistance provided by the strap across the back of his neck.

setting preacher bench curls with incline curls and then supersetting preacher curls (this time using dumbbells) with reverse curls for his forearms.

TIME FOR OTHER PURSUITS

Departing from the six-day-a-week program that he followed earlier in his career, Coe now follows a four-day approach, Monday through Thursday, and takes three days off from exercise. He has found that this works well for him. He also does some running—as fast as he can for a half-mile, not jogging—for increased muscularity.

Obviously, a routine in which every body part is exercised with twenty to thirty sets of varying exercises has to take time. His workouts take about two hours. He can do them in two hours because he trains alone and wastes no time in conversation or waiting for someone else to finish with the equipment.

Does this mean that Boyer Coe is a self-centered beach boy, who just lives to cultivate his muscles? Far from it. He does his exercising from six to eight o'clock in the morning, then cleans up and opens his Body-Masters gym at nine. He puts in a full twelve-hour day instructing others and taking care of the myriad

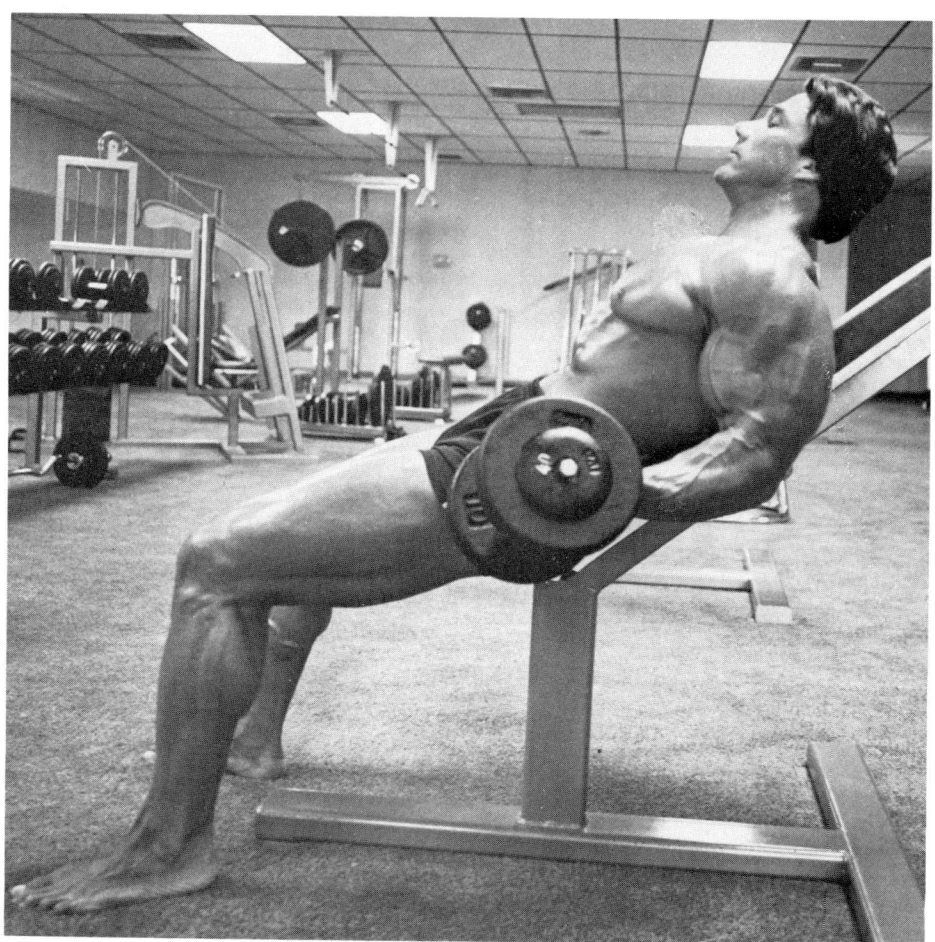

INCLINE BENCH DUMBBELL CURLS, graphically illustrated by this picture of Coe in action, are effective muscle builders.

aspects of his burgeoning food supplement business. Coe gets seven hours of sleep a night and believes another hour would be ideal, but he finds himself too busy to rest as much as he would like.

Coe enjoys bodybuilding and feels that it has been intrinsically good for him, the winning of best-built-man titles aside. He tries to repay the sport by acting as an emissary, speaking before civic groups and other organizations. He started an exercise program for the Louisiana state prison and another for the Louisiana state school for the deaf. He also works with the Big Brother association and other groups that help underprivileged children.

Boyer Coe's pet peeve is that the general public doesn't understand bodybuilding. The public only sees the end result—a powerfully developed man displaying his muscles before an audience—and fails to appreciate the years of athletic training, sacrifice, and mental and physical discipline that are required to mold a champion.

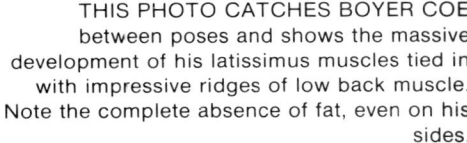

THIS PHOTO CATCHES BOYER COE between poses and shows the massive development of his latissimus muscles tied in with impressive ridges of low back muscle. Note the complete absence of fat, even on his sides.

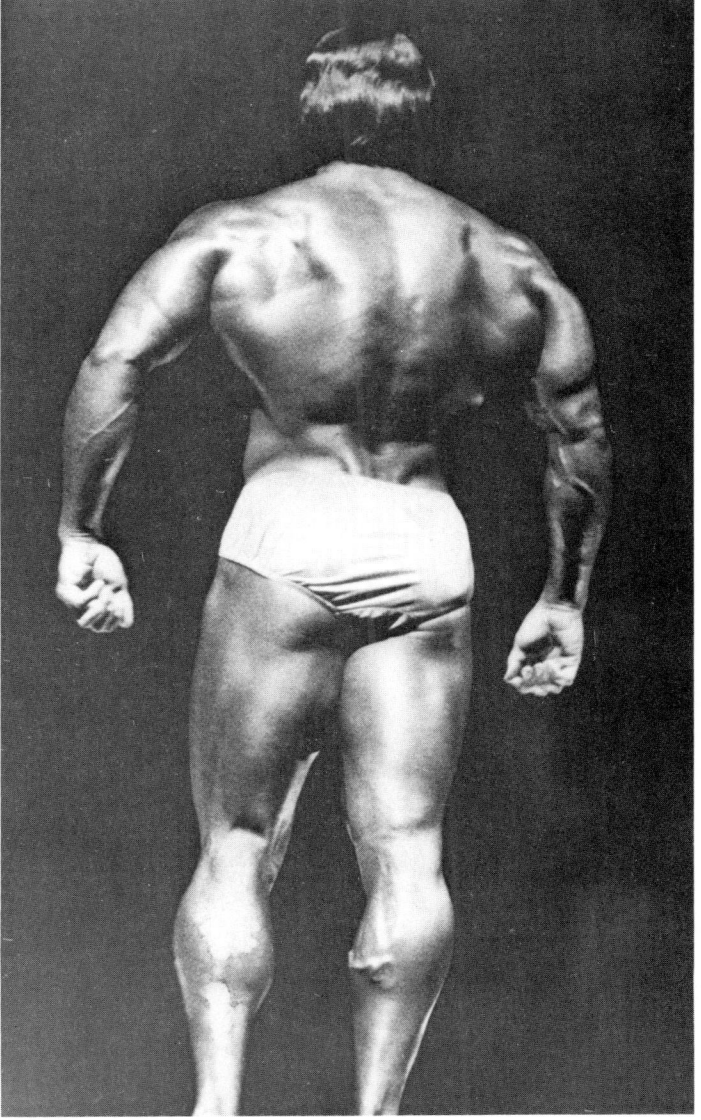

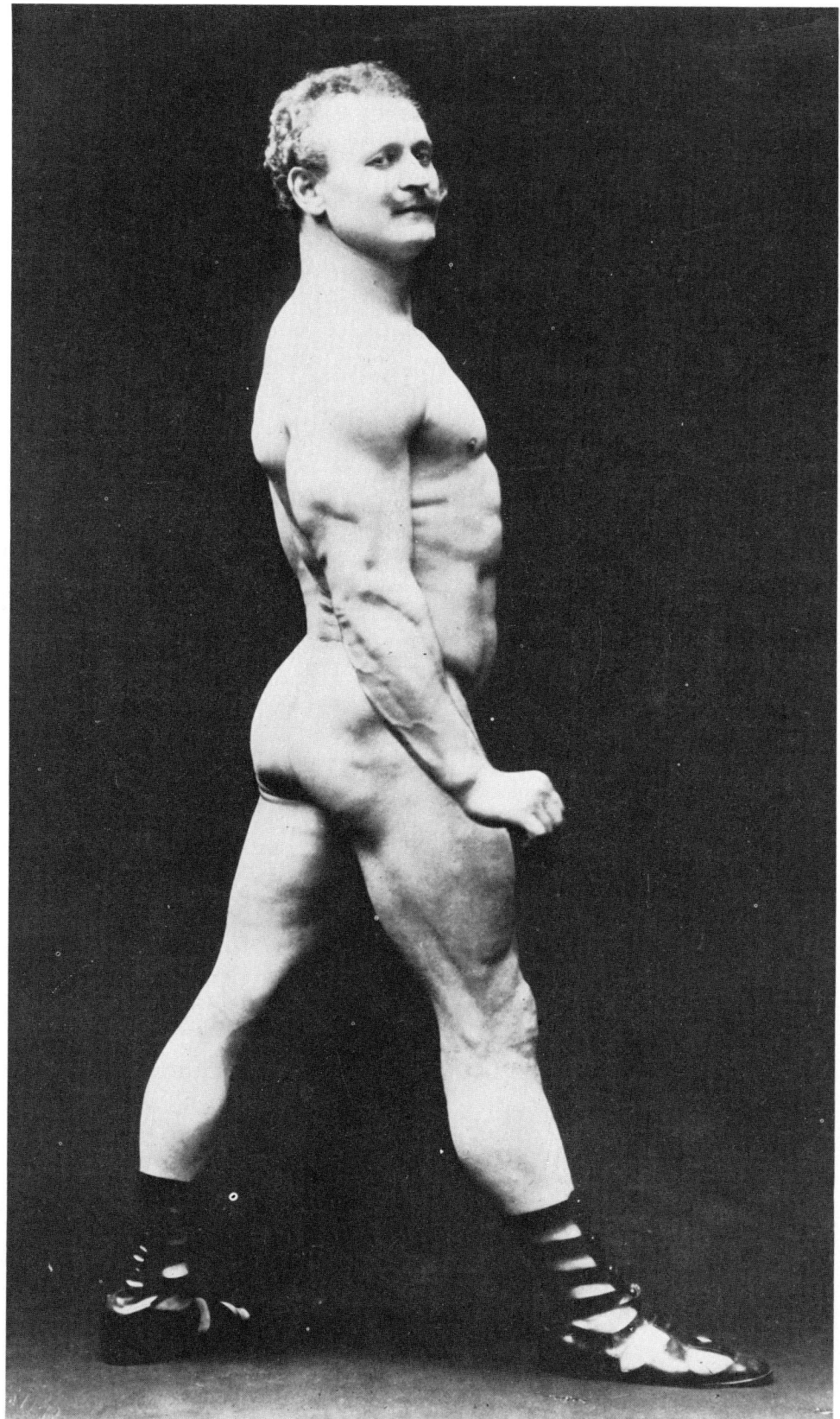

EUGEN SANDOW, the stage name of Prussian strongman Frederick Mueller, was the first man to gain fame and fortune primarily as a result of a superbly developed physique. Sandow's powerful right arm, shown to advantage in the photo, raised 269 pounds in the "bent press" lift.

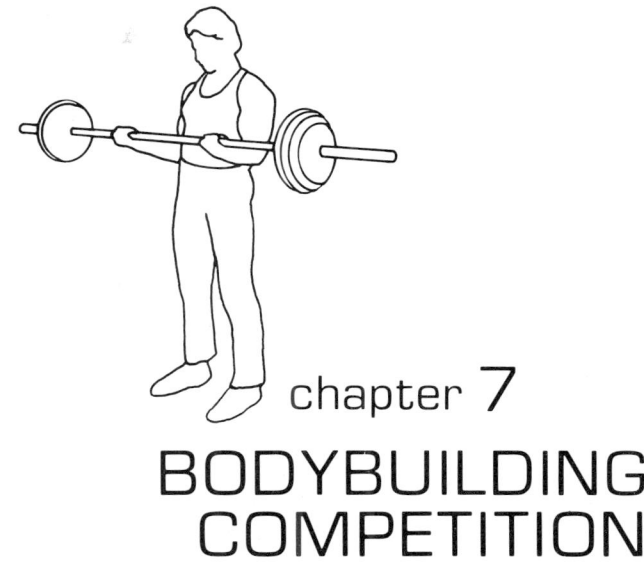

chapter 7

BODYBUILDING COMPETITION

The earliest displays of well-muscled physiques were coincidental with competition in such sports as weight lifting, wrestling, and gymnastics. Training for weight lifting developed the most muscle, so it isn't surprising that presentations of physique display and best-built-man contests evolved with and from this elemental strength sport.

THE FIRST "BODYBUILDER"

The first man to gain international fame and fortune primarily as a result of physique display was Eugen Sandow—a stage name taken by Frederick Mueller, who was born in Koenigsberg, East Prussia, April 2, 1867. Early in his athletic career, the young Sandow participated in weight

lifting, wrestling, and gymnastics, first gaining stature as a leading strongman by defeating two well-known professionals, Charles Sampson and Franz Bienkowski (known as "Cyclops"), in feats of lifting, bar-bending, and chain-breaking.

In his act, Sandow performed a number of spectacular feats, including walking across the stage supporting a pony (about 350 pounds) overhead with one arm (though much of the animal's weight was supported on Sandow's neck and shoulders). He lifted a large barbell that had two massive gloves on the ends, raising it with his right arm in a lift called the bent press. In this lift, the barbell is held at the center of the handle with one hand, the upper arm braced along the lifter's side. Then the lifter leans away from the weight, which straightens his arm. As his arm reaches an almost straight position, he pushes to fully lock the arm and then shifts his weight into a semi-squat position. Finally, he rises to hold the barbell overhead with one arm.

As Sandow performed this maneuver, it would seem evident to the audience that the globes were hollow, and the spectators would begin to wonder if his performance was faked. Then he would set the barbell down, and the globes would open to reveal a small person curled up in each. Everyone has an idea what a person weighs—even a small one—so it was obvious that the total weight of the metal bar, globes, and people had to be in the vicinity of 250 pounds. Using iron weights, Sandow officially lifted 269 pounds in the right arm bent press in 1891. The feat was especially impressive in relation to his size, which was 186 pounds at a height of just under 5'8".

Sandow also was exceptionally agile. He performed standing back somersaults while holding a pair of heavy dumbbells (claimed to weigh 56 pounds each). But it was Sandow's superb physique that set him apart. After performing a few spectacular strength feats, he would mesmerize audiences by posing his powdered white body against a black background, appearing as a living statue.

Strength historian David P. Willoughby, in his book *The Super Athletes*, wrote that "it was Sandow, more than any performer who had preceded him, who raised feats of strength out of the grunt-and-groan category and made them spectacular and entertaining. He was enabled to do this largely by reason of his remarkable physique, in which was combined versatile strength with panther-like grace and agility."

So appealing a personality was Sandow, and so great was his stage presence, that he was able to tour Britain, Europe, South Africa, Australia, and the United States for extended engagements. Willoughby reported that Sandow received $3,500 a week for appearances at the Trocadero Theater in Chicago, a fabulous remuneration at the time. Sandow's promoter at the Trocadero was Florenz—The Great—Ziegfeld.

Sandow's inspiration prompted thousands of young men to take up dumbbells around the turn of the century. He operated a highly successful School of Physical Culture in London and was named "Instructor by Appointment to His Majesty, George V."

CHARLES ATLAS

After Sandow, several professionals capitalized on their muscular development, one of the most noteworthy being Angelo Siciliano, better known as Charles Atlas. Atlas had been chosen "America's most perfectly developed man" in a contest sponsored by Bernarr Macfadden's *Physical Culture* magazine. If he were to have stood alongside any of the modern winners of major physique contests, Atlas would have resembled a beginner more than a winner, but his pleasingly proportioned body, though not notable for muscular development, proved an effective attention-getter for the system of free-hand exercises he sold as "Dynamic Tension." Atlas retained an impressive appearance and superior physical fitness into his seventies, mainly by jogging and using some of his favorite free-hand exercises, such as push-ups.

THE JOHN GRIMEK ERA

Representative and well-organized physique contests began to proliferate in the early 1940s, a Mr. America contest having been held in conjunction with the national Amateur Athletic Union weight lifting championships of 1939. These were formalized contests with standard methods for evaluating contestants, who lined up alongside one another and performed individual muscle displays before a panel of judges.

With the 1940 AAU Mr. America contest, there arrived on the scene the first man since Sandow to thoroughly dominate the field. His name: John C. Grimek, a member of the 1936 Olympic weight lifting team, one of the world's all-around strongest men, and a man who had been training as much for power as for bodybuilding. But Grimek's destiny was bodybuilding for, like Sandow, he had an indefinable quality beyond superb muscular development that set him apart. In pictures, Grimek's massiveness and proportions are apparent, but it isn't possible to visualize the surprising grace and fluidity of motion that this ruggedly constructed man possessed. Grimek, like Sandow, did not have the advantages of more recent developments in apparatus and the sophisticated dietary approaches used by modern bodybuilders, but he had the great natural advantages of extreme mesomorphy and a high-octane metabolism. In his youth, when he was building the foundation for a physique that dominated an era, his family was so poor during a severe economic depression, he told me, that for a time he subsisted on bread and coffee!

When he won his first Mr. America contest in 1940, Grimek weighed only 183 pounds. He had attempted to reduce his weight to the 181-pound weight lifting class but missed by two pounds. So he competed in the national championships as a heavyweight and placed third behind his protege Steve Stanko, a powerful 225-pounder, and equally large Louis Abele, the two best heavyweight lifters in the world at the time.

It was in the Mr. America contest that Grimek came into his own. He was an easy winner. And he won again the next year, 1941, at more than 200 pounds of splendidly proportioned muscle, passing up the weight lifting competition and specializing in bodybuilding. (Incidentally, Grimek's friend Stanko suffered an attack of phlebitis and gave up lifting competition in 1941. He turned to less stressful bodybuilding exercises and won the AAU Mr. America title in 1944. The first man to total 1,000 pounds on the three Olympic lifts, Stanko also won the first Mr. Universe contest in 1947.)

After Grimek's two victories, the AAU passed a rule that a man could win the Mr. America title only once. Grimek then "retired" from competition at 31 and devoted himself to his work as an editor of *Strength & Health* magazine, giving an occasional exhibition, coaching younger men in bodybuilding, and raising his growing family. He was twice persuaded to return to competition, however, once to face handsome young Steve Reeves in the Mr. Universe contest of 1948 and again to meet the challenge of another young Mr. America, Clarence Ross, in the Mr. U.S.A. contest of 1949. After turning back the challenges of Reeves and Ross, Grimek finally did retire from competition, though he never stopped bodybuilding and retained an incredibly muscular and well-proportioned physique past the age of 65.

FAMOUS BODYBUILDERS

Since the Grimek era, there have been increasing numbers of exceptionally well-built men contending for the top physique titles. Without attempting to compile an exhaustive list, some of the most noteworthy were Reeves, Ross, Larry Scott, Boyer Coe, Frank Zane, Ken Waller, Reg Park of England, Franco Columbu of Italy, Serge Nubret of France, and Sergio Oliva, a transplanted Cuban. Only a few, however, have been as dominant as San-

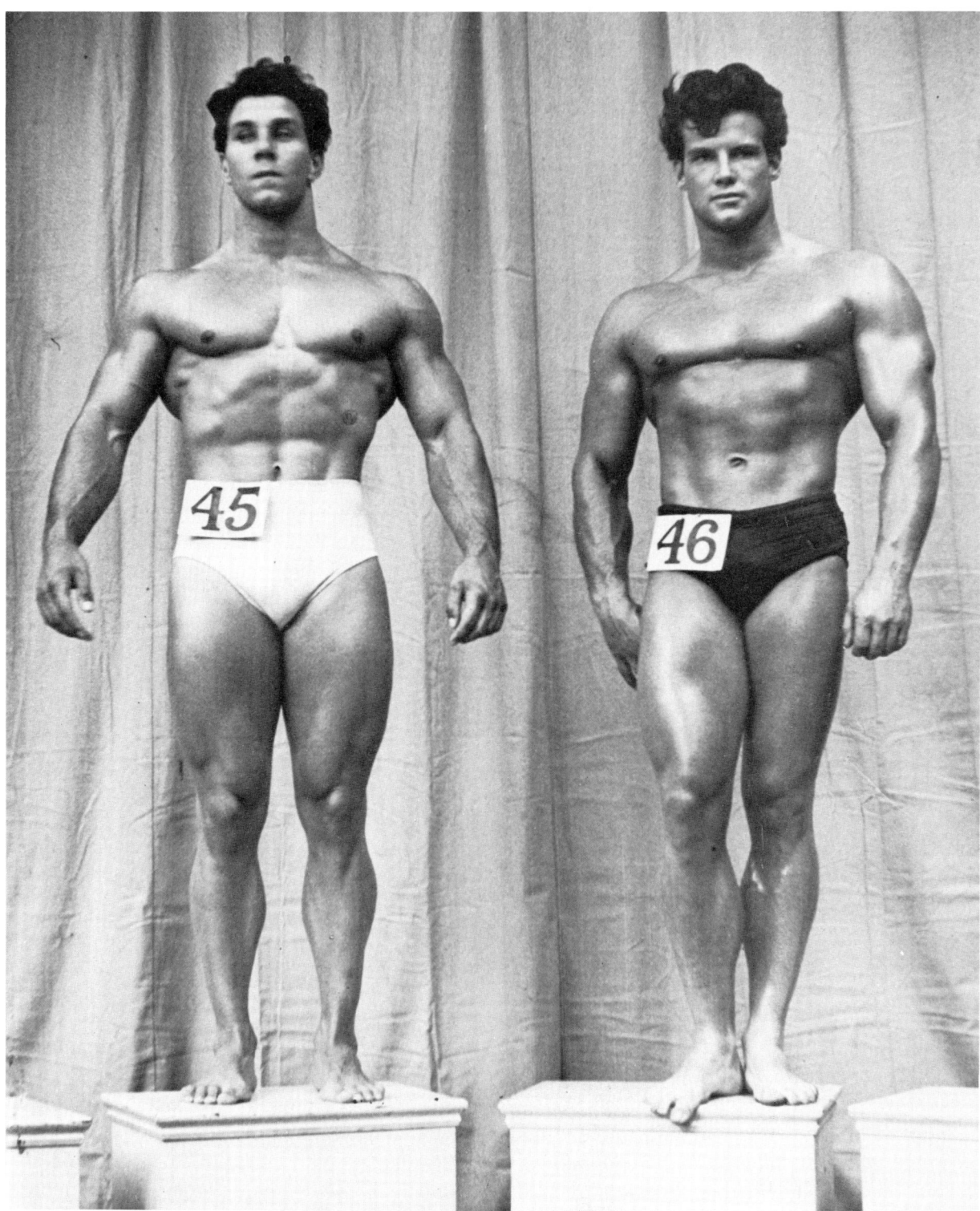

AN INTERESTING COMPARISON of two all-time greats in bodybuilding shows Reg Park of England *(left)* and Steve Reeves of the U.S.A. Superbly muscled six-footers, both won Mr. Universe titles and went on to play strongman roles in popular motion pictures. (Photo courtesy *Strength & Health* magazine)

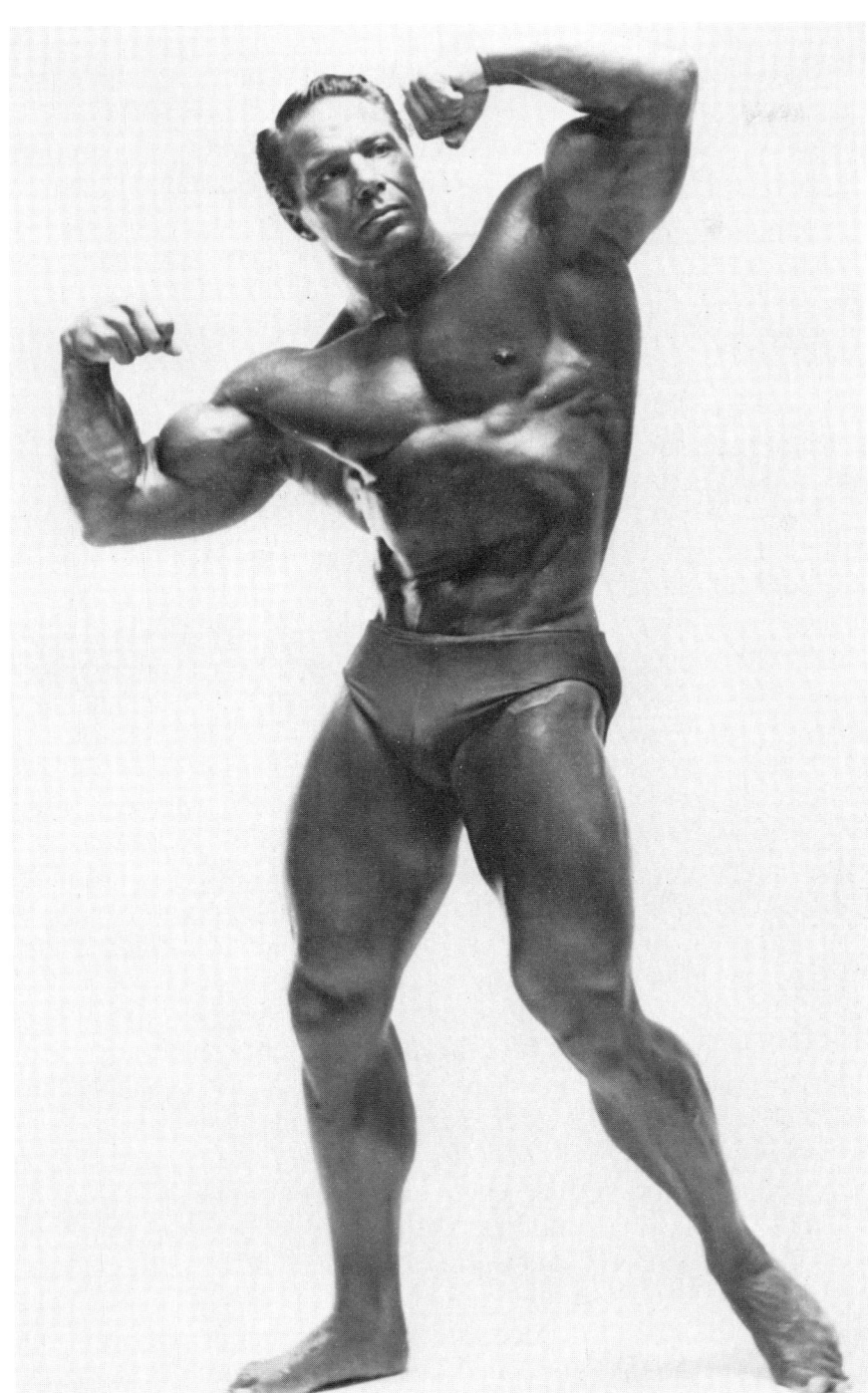

BILL PEARL, an outstanding amateur wrestler before he concentrated on bodybuilding, dominated the sport over an unusually long time span. He won the Mr. America contest in 1953 and a final Mr. Universe title in 1971.

dow and Grimek over extended time spans.

Bill Pearl

One man who did dominate for years was Bill Pearl, who won the Mr. America title in 1953 at 22 and a final Mr. Universe contest in 1971 when he was 41 (only the AAU Mr. America contest bars previous winners from re-entering). In his final contest, Pearl outscored a quality field that included Sergio Oliva, Reg Park, and Frank Zane, all winners of top titles at various times.

Early in his career, Pearl had divided his athletic interests between bodybuilding and wrestling, winning the 13th Naval District championship and finishing as runner-up in the heavyweight class in the 1952 Pacific Northwest Olympic tryouts while serving in the United States Navy. Once he focused on bodybuilding, however, Pearl knew where his real interest lay, and in addition to becoming an all-time great as a competitor he also became one of the really top-flight instructors in the field. Pearl, like Grimek, managed to remain a private person, a devoted family man, despite the demands of his Pasadena gym, a related "Physical Fitness Architects" business, and occasional personal appearances to give exhibitions of strongman stunts and posing, *a la* Sandow.

Arnold Schwarzenegger

The next dominant figure in bodybuilding, Arnold Schwarzenegger, was the antithesis of reserved men such as Grimek and Pearl, whose only public consisted of the sport's aficionados. Schwarzenegger, who moved quickly from Mr. World and Mr. Universe victories to six straight triumphs in the Mr. Olympia contest before retiring from competition at 29, became a self-assured public figure.

Taking a leaf from Steve Reeves's book, he gained parts in movies and television shows and was featured in a film on the subject of bodybuilding, "Pumping Iron." Unlike the more restrained Reeves, however, Schwarzenegger was aggressively extroverted, becoming an ambassador for bodybuilding to the general public, who at best had barely heard of the activity before seeing Arnold on television "talk shows" and reading about him in periodicals with wide general circulation.

A PROLIFERATION OF CONTESTS

Although the Amateur Athletic Union (AAU) had initiated physique competition as an adjunct to weight lifting contests, the activity grew at a greater rate and aroused more public interest than lifting. Partly because AAU weight lifting and physique competition were closely tied to the commercial enterprises of Bob Hoffman's York Barbell Company and Strength & Health Publishing Company, rival organizations arose to sponsor best-built-man contests. The best-known and most successful of these was the International Federation of Bodybuilders (IFBB), headed by Ben Weider and promoted by his brother, Joe, head of the Weider Barbell Company and publisher of *Muscle Builder/Power* magazine. A third such organization, the World Body Building Guild (WBBG), was formed by Dan Lurie, a former bodybuilding champion and television strongman, who headed the Lurie Barbell Company and published *Muscle Training Illustrated* magazine.

Outside the United States, the British National Amateur Body Building Association (NABBA) staged an annual Mr. Universe contest of exceptionally high quality in addition to national contests. Because NABBA had no commercial ties, victories in its Mr. Universe contests were

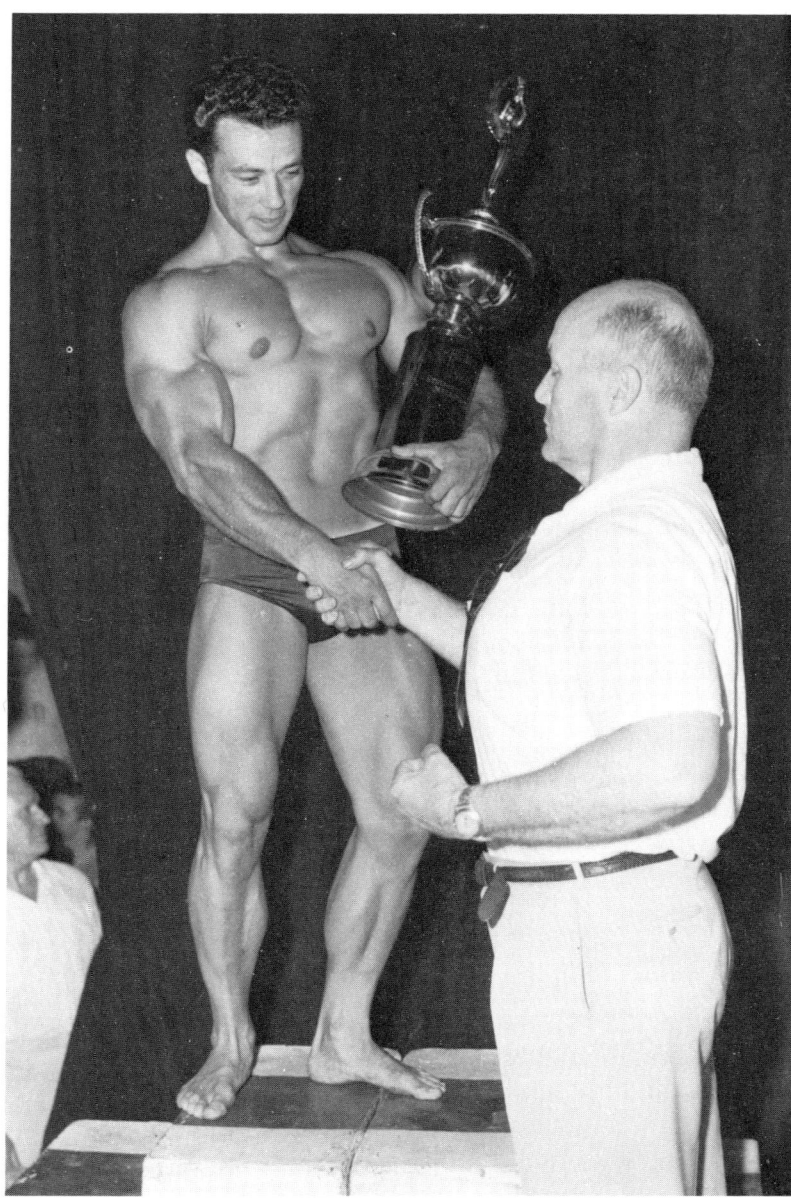

BOB HOFFMAN, shown clowning for a photographer while presenting the winner's trophy to 1952 Mr. America Jim Park, has been a patron of both bodybuilding and weight lifting, throwing most of his resources behind the strength sport. Hoffman built an empire consisting of the York Barbell Company, Hoffman Food Supplements, and Strength & Health Publishing Company. He coached several victorious Olympic and world weightlifting championship teams. (Photo courtesy *Strength & Health* magazine)

especially valued by contestants, who considered them evidence of excellence in the opinion of unbiased experts.

The Pros and Cons

The commercial tie-in of the York, Weider, and Lurie organizations with the governing bodies of the various associations that sponsor and control the sport of bodybuilding has had both positive and negative aspects. On the positive side, these commercial firms had the funds to promote and develop the sport, which clearly has had a beneficial effect on the health and physical fitness consciousness of countless thousands, probably millions, of people. They also have done much to develop bodybuilding as a sport. Hoffman promoted and supported weight lifting to a greater extent than bodybuilding, but he did encourage bodybuilding and sponsored contestants in that sport as well. Joe and Ben Weider threw their full energies into the development of bodybuilding and succeeded in making the IFBB a major international sports organization. The untiring efforts of Ben, a patient and dedicated organizer, were complemented by the enthusiasm and promotional activities of his brother, Joe, surely the world's number one bodybuilding fan.

On the negative side, there is an overlapping proliferation of contests that diminishes the significance of winning major titles, which are duplicated by the various governing bodies. For example, the AAU, IFBB, and WBBG all select Mr. America and Mr. World titlists. The IFBB and NABBA both hold Mr. Universe contests. These are all top quality contests, and the winners are worthy titleholders, but it certainly seems desirable to sort these events out so that only one Mr. America, one Mr. World, and one Mr. Universe are chosen each year. Unfortunately, the business rivalries and egos involved have prevented the various organizations from getting together and eliminating the confusion.

Another negative aspect of the rivalry has been that competing bodybuilders associated in one way or another with one of the organizations tend to get unfair treatment from the others. There is no question that pre-contest publicity affects the contestant's chances of winning or placing in a physique contest, and the magazines heavily publicize their favorites. I make that statement as a person who has judged both AAU and IFBB contests and tries his utmost to score the contestants according to established judging standards, as I think most of the other judges do as well. It is difficult, however, not to be influenced by the fact that you have seen a hundred pictures of one contestant, a half-dozen of another, and are seeing a third man perhaps for the first time.

Where to Get Contest Information

Despite certain drawbacks imposed by the rivalries, if you are interested in bodybuilding competition, you will have to affiliate yourself with the organization that sponsors the contest(s) you are hopeful of winning. Information can be obtained from:

Amateur Athletic Union of
  the United States
3400 West 86th Street
Indianapolis, IN 46268

International Federation of
  BodyBuilders
2875 Bates Road
Montreal, Ouebec
Canada H3S 1B7

World Body Building Guild
1665 Utica Avenue
Brooklyn, NY 11234

WHAT JUDGES LOOK FOR

Physique competition is based on a number of elements that are taken into consideration by the judges. One, obviously, is muscular development. This means all the muscles. A man does not win a major contest if he has only big arms, shoulders, and chest muscles, with underdeveloped legs. As the competition gets tougher, judges look for fine points— the muscles of the lower back, the forearms, the neck.

Another element might be termed muscularity, or definition. This is simply an absence of fat covering the muscles. Some bodybuilders become so defined that they literally look like human anatomical charts, clearly showing details of the external obliques, serratus, sartorius, brachialis, and other muscles that cannot be seen through the skin of non-body-builders, either because they are not well developed or are hidden by a layer of fat. (This layer of fat may be very thin, incidentally, and quite normal for a well-conditioned athlete. A bodybuilder in contest condition is trained down as "fine" as a muscular wrestler who has reduced 20 pounds to enter a specific class.)

Bodybuilders also are judged on harmonious proportions and symmetry. Their muscular development should be in harmony with their bone structure, and no body part should stand out more than any other. The judge asks himself, "Is this man's back as well developed and defined as his chest? Are his forearms as well developed as his biceps and triceps? Are his calves in proportion with his thighs?"

Beyond harmonious muscular develop-ment and definition, an experienced judge will consider the contestant's bone structure and skin texture. When contestants are evenly matched, almost intangible differences may make the difference. Does the contestant look fit? Does he move with the grace of an athlete? Is he confident and relaxed or in a constant state of muscular tension? In the final analysis, neat hair and appropriate posing trunks may make the fraction of a point difference between the first and second place man!

The only way truly to understand how physique contests are conducted is to attend one or more. This, along with obtaining official rule books, will show you how the veteran contestants present themselves and give you an idea of what the judges are looking for.

SHOWING BOTH MUSCLE MASS
AND clear-cut definition, Boyer Coe's
physique is the product of hard
training on a carefully organized
exercise program and a well-planned
diet, including supplements.

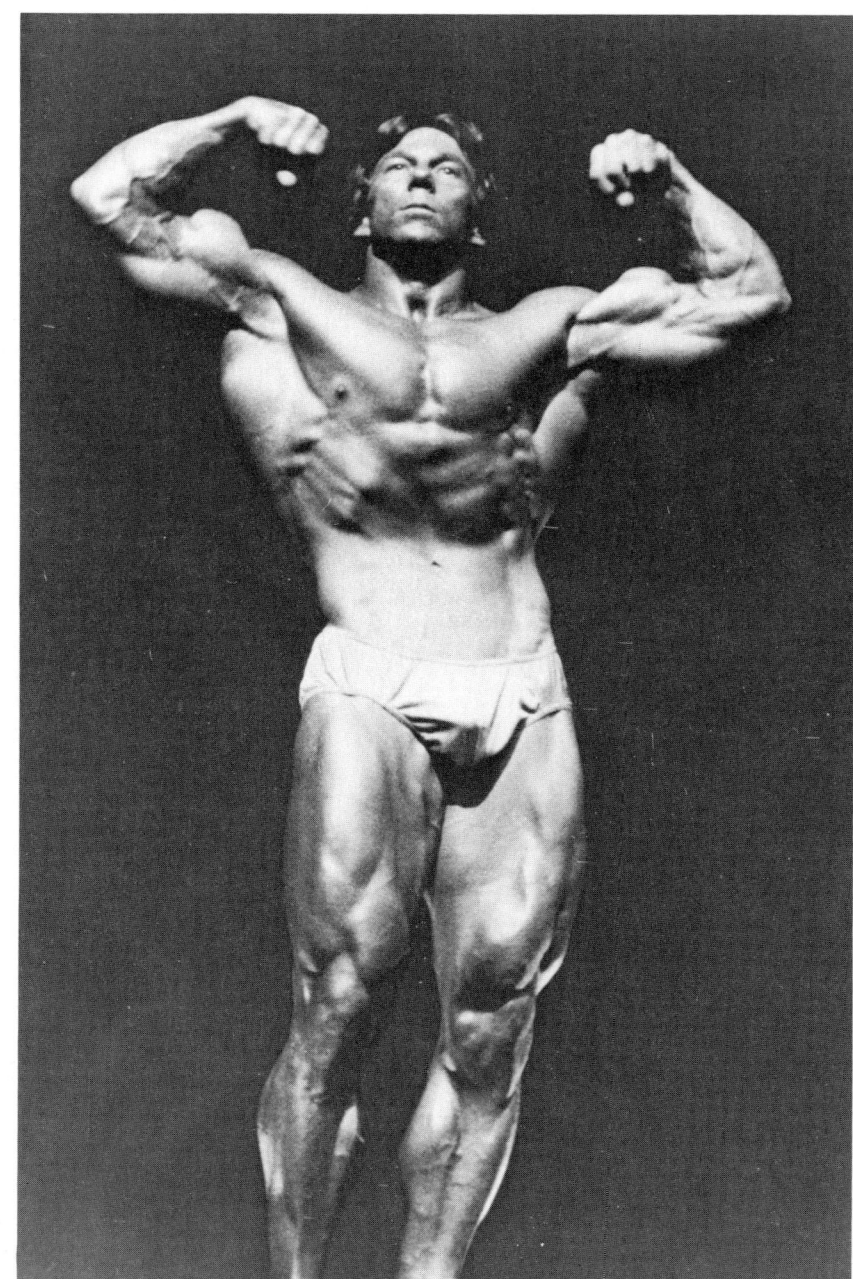

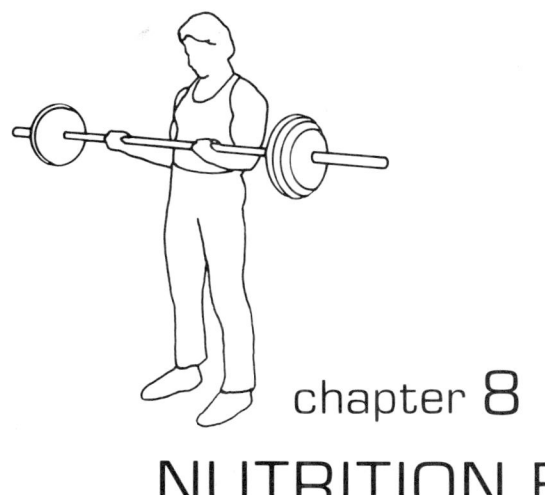

chapter 8

NUTRITION FOR BODYBUILDING

Many leading bodybuilders consider nutrition as important as exercise in their programs. Certainly adhering to a bodybuilder's diet requires more discipline than is required to exercise. The exercise program takes from two to four hours a day, three to six days a week, while the serious bodybuilder must adhere to his diet twenty-four hours a day, seven days a week.

It is difficult to say how much careful attention to diet has to do with building muscle, but it certainly has a great deal to do with muscularity (muscle definition, or visibility beneath the skin). The modern bodybuilder does not have any more muscles than the best men had twenty and thirty years ago, but he is better able to display what he has because his diet removes almost all vestiges of subcutaneous fat. In fact, so devoid of normal fat reserves is the modern bodybuilder that he is not really at his physical peak for performance at the same time that he is at his peak for appearing in a physique contest. If he has timed his training and diet correctly, the bodybuilder will have no reserves left when he appears before the judges. This tends to weaken a man somewhat, but it produces an appearance of extreme muscularity.

DIET ESSENTIALS

There are many individual variations in bodybuilders' approaches to diet, but they share the following general elements:

    High protein intake
    Low carbohydrate intake
    Inclusion of supplements

To increase muscle-building protein intake, bodybuilders include eggs and lean meats in their diets. Their scanty carbohydrate intake comes from fruits and vegetables, and they eliminate or greatly restrict intake of refined flour and sugar. Most bodybuilders consume relatively large quantities of salads for the roughage, vitamins, and minerals contained in lettuce and similar greens. Because their diet is overbalanced on the protein side, bodybuilders also must drink a great deal of water. That is because it takes about seven times as much water to metabolize protein as it take to metabolize fat or carbohydrate. Kidney damage can result from a high protein diet with restricted fluid intake.

Incidentally, there is no scientific evidence showing that cholesterol from meat, eggs, and milk products is harmful to a person who is metabolically normal and vigorously active. John Balik, a self-educated nutritionist who has studied the scientific literature on nutrition from a physical culturist's point of view, believes that eggs, milk, and meat are harmless to an active bodybuilder as long as he avoids refined sugar. Balik points out that fats associated with meat are good energy sources and also sources from which the body makes natural hormones.

Boyer Coe, Mr. America and Mr. Universe winner and one of the outstanding instructors among best-built-man champions, recommends rare meat as a good protein source because it digests more rapidly than well-cooked meat. On the other hand, Coe does not recommend adding raw eggs to protein drinks. Because raw eggs are hard to digest, Coe recommends that they be soft boiled and then blended into the drink.

As to supplements, Coe recommends desiccated liver for stamina and energy, vitamin C, the B vitamins, and vitamin E

(to boost the oxygen-carrying capacity of the blood). Balik also recommends liver tablets and at least a gram of vitamin C with bioflavinoids daily. Wheat germ oil, especially Viobin brand, is the source of vitamin E recommended by Balik, who cautions that it should not be taken on an empty stomach.

Both Coe and Balik stress the superiority of protein supplements from egg, milk, and meat sources because of their proper amino acid balance. Coe has taken the step of developing his own Amino Bond Gold brand of liquid, predigested protein, made from animal sources. This supplement is hydrolized into the amino acids used by the body for muscle building. There are many protein supplements available, so it is important to determine their amino acid composition in order to obtain the most nutritionally useful "essential" components. Some supplements have a high protein content but lack the proper mix of essential and nonessential amino acids.

THE COMPETITION DIET

In preparing for bodybuilding competition, Boyer Coe recommends eating small quantities of food about six times a day, at regular intervals. He says you should never stuff yourself, but never allow yourself to become hungry. Coe believes that diet is more important for building muscle with definition than varying the numbers of repetitions and sets of exercises. He also points out that acquiring muscularity takes time; it can't be done by dieting strictly for the last two or three weeks before a contest, which he feels will leave a person looking drawn, with diminished muscle size.

Coe suggests a controlled diet for at least three months before a contest to allow your system to adjust to new eating habits. It would include reduction of car-

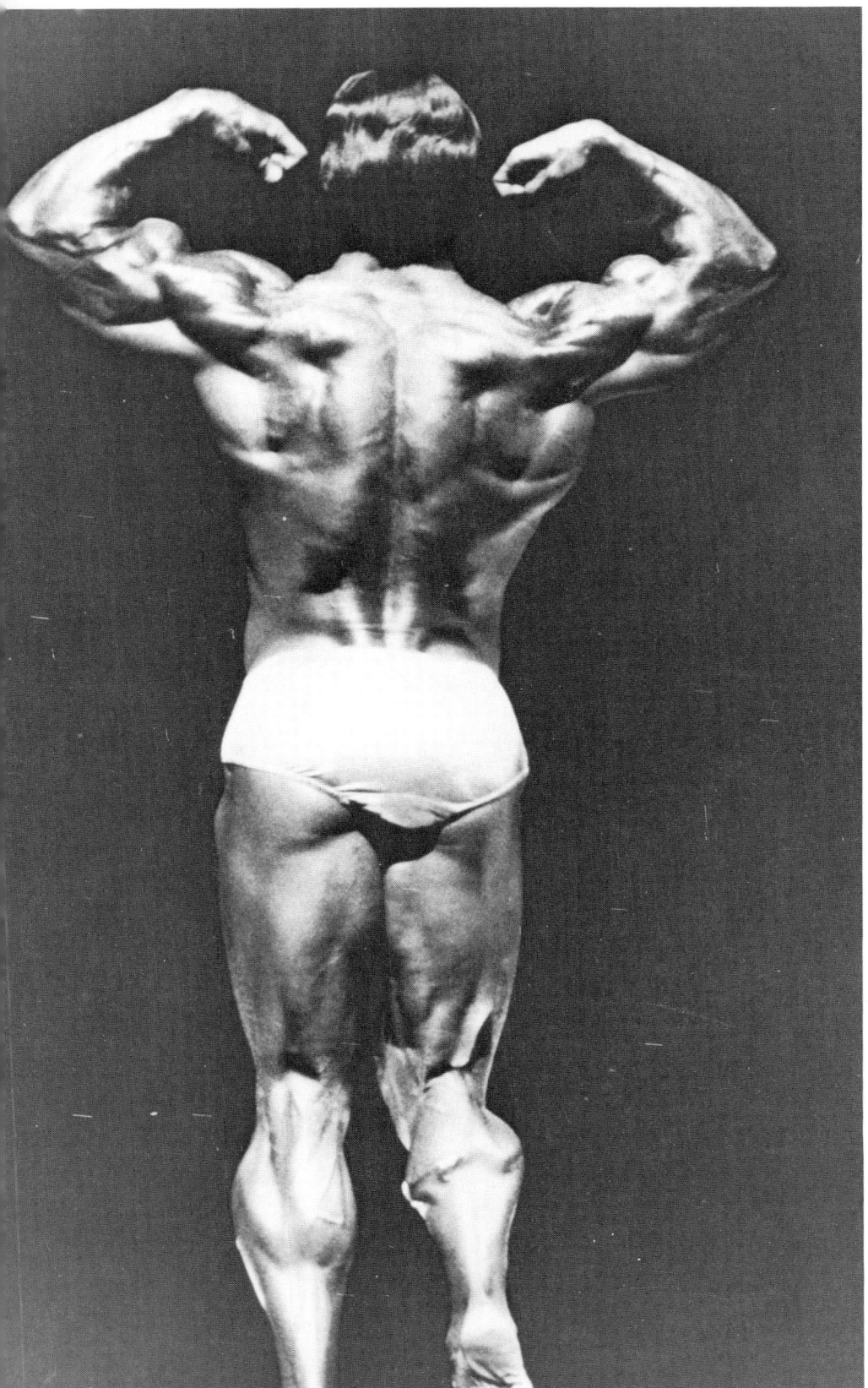

A HIGH-PROTEIN DIET, supplemented with vitamins, helped Boyer Coe keep his body free of fat as he built muscle with heavy exercise.

bohydrate intake, including vegetable sources of carbohydrates. To compensate for nutritional deficiencies that could result, he recommends vitamin supplements. He believes milk should be eliminated from a bodybuilder's diet six to eight weeks before a contest because he feels it has a tendency to deposit a thin layer of fat just under the skin. When eliminating milk, he recommends taking a calcium supplement. He also recommends taking a kelp supplement to help reduce body fat. The following diet is one Coe has found effective in acquiring muscular density for competition:

Breakfast: Steak and eggs; 1 slice of 7-grain bread; 2 ounces of Amino Bond Gold hydrolized protein in 6 ounces of fresh orange juice; 2,000 mg of vitamin C; 800 i.u. of vitamin E; 15 desiccated liver tablets; 5 kelp tablets; 1,000 mg of choline.

Mid-morning: 2 ounces of Amino Bond Gold in 6 ounces of fresh orange juice.

Noon: Steak or fish; 2 ounces of Amino Bond Gold; 2,000 mg of vitamin C; 800 i.u. of vitamin E; 15 desiccated liver tablets; 5 kelp tablets; 1,000 mg of choline.

Mid-afternoon: Small steak or can of tuna; 1 ounce of Amino Bond Gold.

Supper: Large steak (2-lb); 2 ounces of Amino Bond Gold; 2,000 mg of vitamin C; 800 i.u. of vitamin E; 15 desiccated liver tablets; 1,000 mg of choline.

Bedtime: 2 ounces of Amino Bond Gold; 2,000 mg of vitamin C; 800 i.u. of vitamin E; 15 desiccated liver tablets; 5 kelp tablets; 1,000 mg choline.

In addition to the supplements listed as taken regularly, Coe also added calcium, B vitamins, and vitamin A to his pre-contest diet from time to time. His regular diet stresses beef, liver, chicken, fish, eggs, cheese, vegetables, and fruits. He continues to supplement his diet with his own brand of desiccated liver and yeast tablets, as well as vitamins E and C, kelp, choline, inositol, and minerals even when not preparing specifically for a contest. Instead of mixing Amino Bond Gold protein supplement with orange juice, he may vary his between-meals protein snack by mixing the supplement with whipping cream.

As you can see, championship bodybuilding preparation requires more than dietary discipline; it also calls for a budget that permits purchase of high protein natural foods and large quantities of supplements.

Weight-gain Drink

Many bodybuilders are less concerned about getting into contest condition than about gaining muscle size. One way of boosting solid weight gain is by adding a weight-gain drink that contains ample protein and carbohydrates. Here is an example of a drink that can be prepared in a blender:

24 ounces of milk
½-cup high quality protein supplement (milk or egg source or hydrolized amino acids)
4 to 6 slightly boiled eggs
1 ripe banana
a generous scoop of ice cream

The weight-gain drink can be consumed at various times over the course of a day. It may be necessary to re-blend it after it has been sitting in a refrigerator for a period of time. A supplement such as a weight-gain drink can be added to a normal balanced diet and should enhance muscle growth for a young man on a bodybuilding program. For that matter, such a supplement also would promote solid weight gain for an underweight woman who was practicing bodybuilding exercises. If someone were to take such a supplement and not exercise, however, the likely result would be to put on fat.

PHYSICAL FITNESS DIET

For a person who uses bodybuilding as an aspect of total physical fitness, nutritional extremes should be avoided. Since a body free of all subcutaneous fat is unnatural, total avoidance of carbohydrates seems unnecessary. There is medical evidence, (as well as the experience of physical culturists) to suggest that consuming large quantities of refined sugars is unhealthy; so obtaining carbohydrates from fruits and vegetables appears to be a good idea.

A sensible diet would include foods from the following groups:

- Leafy green vegetables and yellow vegetables.
- Citrus fruits, tomatoes, raw cabbage, and salad greens.
- Milk and such milk products as cheese and cottage cheese.
- Eggs, meat, poultry, fish, and legumes.
- Potatoes and similar root foods.
- Bread and cereal.
- Butter or margarine or vegetable oil.

All of the important nutritional elements are available from the foregoing food groups. In addition, there can be no harm in taking a multi-vitamin supplement, and other supplements are worth experimenting with to see if they improve physical performance or a sense of well-being.

Anabolic Steroids

While on the subject of supplements, it is appropriate to consider the use of anabolic steroids, though these really come under the heading of drugs. Whereas bodybuilding can be a health-building activity when coupled with sound nutri-

tion, adequate rest, and other diverse interests, the use of anabolic steroids shows how any sport can become perverted by a win-at-any-cost attitude.

Anabolic steroids are chemical analogs of male hormones, and they are used medically to treat deficiencies in aged people whose natural production of hormones has become impaired. A careful review of the effects of these drugs by leading scientists has led to anabolic steroids being labeled "probably" effective in the treatment of senile and postmenopausal osteoporosis, providing they are given as an adjunct to a controlled diet and physical therapy.

The anabolic steroids are known to have dangerous side effects. They affect glucose tolerance and liver function and are suspected of contributing to cancer of the prostate gland.

Despite these drawbacks, many bodybuilders and other athletes in sports requiring strength and power believe them to be "magic pills" that produce miraculous muscle growth. So they take these drugs illicitly, regardless of what long-term harm they may do. Both common sense and medical evidence cry out against the use of anabolic steroids for bodybuilding effect. Medically, there are known dangers, but the ultimate effect of this tampering with the body's normal functioning will not be known for another ten to twenty years, when young men who have taken anabolics indiscriminantly become middle-aged.

Common sense suggests that these drugs are taken to no good purpose since men developed as much muscle in years past when no anabolic steroids were used. Furthermore, improvement in athletic performance and muscularity by champions who refrain from drugs can be attributed to harder, more systematic training, improved equipment, and nutrition.

index